PRAISE FOR *UNDERSTANDING AUTOIMMUNE DISEASE*

"*Understanding Autoimmune Disease: A Therapist's Guide to Invisible Illness* is a groundbreaking and compassionate guide to the psychological realities of living with autoimmune disease and how invisible illness intersects with identity, trauma, and systemic bias. Drawing from her dual perspective as both clinician and patient, Dr. Skoufalos explores medical trauma, diagnostic delay, and the emotional toll of being disbelieved. What if healing isn't about fixing what's broken but remembering what was never lost? And what if the most healing thing a clinician could do is simply believe their patient?"

—NATALIE R. COHEN, PsyD, founder of
Mindwise Psychology, PC

"Dr. Skoufalos writes with both authority and compassion on the topic of autoimmune illness. In this highly accessible book, she integrates a review of the literature and challenges the status quo. She offers new insights and essential skills for mental health professionals working with people with autoimmune illness. A must-read."

—REBECA SCHERMAN, PsyD, clinical psychologist

"*Understanding Autoimmune Disease: A Therapist's Guide to Invisible Illness* is a groundbreaking and deeply compassionate guide for therapists working with clients navigating autoimmune disease. Dr. Skoufalos blends clinical expertise with lived experience to illuminate the often-overlooked emotional and psychological toll of invisible illness. With powerful case examples, nuanced discussions of trauma and practical tools, this book fills a critical gap in mental health care. It's an essential read for any clinician committed to truly seeing and supporting this underserved population."

—LISA ORBÉ-AUSTIN, PhD, licensed psychologist and author of *Own Your Greatness*

———

"*Understanding Autoimmune Disease: A Therapist's Guide to Invisible Illness* is a powerful and compassionate guide that illuminates the emotional challenges of living with an autoimmune disease. As a patient, I recognized my own experiences in the honest exploration of fear, identity shifts and the struggle to be understood. This book offers not just validation, but a path forward toward self-advocacy and reclaiming a sense of empowerment."

—MARISA, a patient living with autoimmune disease

———

UNDERSTANDING AUTOIMMUNE DISEASE

UNDERSTANDING AUTOIMMUNE DISEASE

A THERAPIST'S GUIDE TO INVISIBLE ILLNESS

Nicoletta C. Skoufalos, PhD

Hatherleigh Press, Ltd.

62545 State Highway 10,

Hobart, NY 13788, USA

hatherleighpress.com

UNDERSTANDING AUTOIMMUNE DISEASE

Library of Congress Cataloging-in-Publication Data is available.

ISBN: 978-1-961293-36-6

Printed in the United States

The authorized representative in the EU for product safety and compliance is Catarina Astrom, Blästorpsvägen 14, 276 35 Borrby, Sweden. info@hatherleighpress.com

10 9 8 7 6 5 4 3 2 1

Hatherleigh Press is committed to preserving and protecting the natural resources of the earth. Environmentally responsible and sustainable practices are embraced within the company's mission statement.

Visit us at www.hatherleighpress.com.

CONTENTS

PREFACE

I MET DR. NICOLETTA Skoufalos almost 20 years ago during our freshman year at Fordham University in Lincoln Center. We had an instant connection as we bonded over our love for the Mediterranean and having the privilege of visiting our families in Greece and Italy during the summer. We also connected over our love for the ocean and the sun and how rejuvenating and carefree these experiences made us feel.

Nicoletta soon became my warm, genuine, funny, smart and compassionate Greek sister. We navigated many psychology classes together and have watched one another become clinicians who are passionate about working with people with chronic and often invisible illness. Nicoletta is my go-to referral for people living with autoimmune diseases because I know they will receive the compassionate, well-informed, respectful and loving care they deserve. Being able to call her friend and colleague is a true gift to me.

When Dr. Skoufalos asked me to write the foreword for her book, I was both shocked and honored. This book is truly a labor of love, written with intention, care, and respect while providing important information and critical steps for working with clients in an effective and thoughtful manner. I wish I'd had access to a guide like this during my postdoctoral training or when I initially started my private practice ten years ago.

Dr. Skoufalos has created a masterfully written, timely guide for clinicians working with people experiencing chronic illness. I devoured this book, and to say that I received an education from its content is an understatement! After reading *Understanding Autoimmune Disease: A Therapist's Guide to Invisible Illness*, I feel seen as a human being living with endometriosis as well as supported and challenged as a clinician who works with many clients presenting with an array of invisible illnesses.

As clinicians, we can often feel ill-equipped to work with people who have autoimmune diseases because of a lack of knowledge, training and skill development. Our own biases around invisible illness can also unintentionally harm the therapeutic relationship, resulting in clients feeling invalidated, unheard or gaslit. In this book, Dr. Skoufalos beautifully and skillfully gives us the tools we need to develop our own self-awareness as clinicians working with this population by providing us with helpful self-exploratory questions to challenge our own biases. Nicoletta also provides essential, empirically supported knowledge and research concerning autoimmune diseases to debunk common myths even we clinicians believe about chronic illness—ideas that are simply untrue.

Furthermore, Dr. Skoufalos gives us the concrete skills we need as clinicians to conceptualize, validate, witness and help alchemize our clients' experiences so that they can live a life with joy, integrity and meaning.

Dr. Skoufalos' comprehensive approach to care for her clients really shines through in this handbook, as she recounts specific client's experiences, takes intersections of identity into consideration by validating how racism, sexism and classism (both in our field and as a larger system) can adversely impact our clients, and how we as clinicians must be avid advocates for systemic change. And finally, Dr. Skoufalos' personal account of her experience with lupus made this work so relatable, personal and connecting. I appreciate this approach as a clinician reading this account because it kept me engaged and yearning to learn more about how to effectively help clients with chronic invisible illness.

Thank you, Dr. Skoufalos, for your vulnerability, openness to sharing your work and for your high level of skill and care. This handbook is such a gift to all of us and I look forward to witnessing the ripple effect this labor of love will have on the lives of all the clients we continue to touch every day!

—Cristina Dorazio, PhD, founder of Unity Psychological Consulting

FOREWORD

A PERSON LIVING WITH an autoimmune disease faces many challenges. Often, the first challenge is getting an accurate diagnosis. It can take too many years, too many tests, too many visits to medical offices, too many and too long hospitalizations before hearing for the first time, "You have an autoimmune disease." A second and simultaneous challenge is often not having the support they need during this long, difficult and painful journey.

With the publication of *Understanding Autoimmune Disease: A Therapist's Guide to Invisible Illness*, Dr. Nicoletta Skoufalos offers an insightful and understandable resource for therapists working with people who are living with chronic autoimmune diseases. Having both the professional experience of treating people living with autoimmune disease and the personal experience of living with lupus herself, Dr. Skoufalos challenges therapists to put assumptions aside to truly listen to their patients with an open mind. While this may seem straightforward, as Dr. Skoufalos documents with well-researched references, this is often not the case.

Throughout this helpful guide, Dr. Skoufalos offers firsthand accounts from patients who have felt invisible, misunderstood, misdiagnosed, ignored or worse in places and with people they put their trust in. She challenges therapists to consider what presumptions or assumptions consciously or unconsciously they can be bringing to the therapist-patient relationship which can cause more harm. She tackles the complex intersection of physical health, trauma, loss and grief people experience with practical strategies for navigating conversations in partnership with patients.

Over the years, I've had the opportunity to hear and learn from Dr. Skoufalos as a speaker at a number of programs. She is warm, thoughtful, open, pragmatic and knowledgeable. She engages with her audience members, often people living with lupus and other autoimmune diseases, with respect and offers information to help give them some agency over their lives which can often feel beyond their control. She extends this same spirit to the clinicians who look to this book as a guide, recognizing that there will be a diversity of approaches and patient responses in each working relationship. Throughout the book, she encourages and educates while bringing empathy based on her own experiences.

It is clear that more and better mental health resources are needed for clinicians treating people living with autoimmune diseases. This is a great start and I am hopeful that this work will grow and become a part of every therapist's training.

—Sue Gloor, Division Vice President, Lupus Foundation of America

THE INVISIBLE ILLNESS

"*You're just tired.*" "*You have too much stress.*" "*You have to change your diet.*" "*Maybe if you exercised more.*" "*You are so dramatic.*" "*We all get tired.*" "*At least it's not cancer.*" "*But you look fine.*"

These are just some of the many comments that people who have **autoimmune diseases** often hear from others when they are expressing how they feel. They may hear these comments from their friends and family, and even from well-meaning doctors, including mental health professionals, who at times may feel desperate to offer help but who do not quite know how. Both books and training on psychotherapy for patients with cancer, cardiac disease and pain management exist, but where are the resources for mental health professionals who work with **autoimmune disease** patients?

This book is the first guide designed for mental health professionals who are working with or want to work with people who live with **autoimmune disease**. There are no books written, less than a handful of articles, and to my knowledge, no training for mental health professionals specifically on how to work with people who have **autoimmune disease**. Perhaps this is a manifestation and example of how people living with **autoimmune disease** often feel invisible.

Autoimmune disease is a type of illness in which one's own immune system, specifically one's own autoantibodies, targets healthy tissues in the body, signaling the body to attack them as if they were foreign or unhealthy, such as a virus or a bacterium. This malfunction of the immune system results in excessive inflammation that can cause problems in the muscular, neurological, endocrine, rheumatological, and hormonal systems of the body. **Autoimmune diseases** are mysterious, not well understood diseases that are partly caused by a genetic predisposition (e.g. isolated gene variants involved in the development of lupus; Lupus Research Alliance, 2023) and triggered by environmental toxins and/or stressors, such as Epstein-Barr infection, trauma, or sustained heightened states of stress. Although in the last decade there has been an increased interest in researching **autoimmune diseases**, funding for this research has historically been significantly less than funding provided for research on other illnesses, such as cancer and HIV (Shomon, 2002). There is some hope that there will be increased interest in better understanding **autoimmune disease** following the emergence of large numbers of people who have developed autoimmune-like symptoms due to long Covid (O'Rourke, 2022). There are treatments for **autoimmune diseases** but there are no cures. **Autoimmune diseases** run in families. They typically present more often in women (80 percent are women according to the Autoimmune Association, 2024), and in some **autoimmune diseases** such as lupus, they specifically appear in women of color (Lupus Foundation of America, 2024). Having one **autoimmune disease** increases one's chances of having other **autoimmune diseases** (Ge, Li, Wang, & Zuo, 2020).

INVISIBLE ILLNESS AND THE JOURNEY OF INVISIBILITY

This group of illnesses is often called "invisible illness" because outside (and sometimes despite) blood tests and imaging exams, the symptoms and the suffering of the person is typically not visible to others. Examples of such illnesses are lupus, rheumatoid arthritis, multiple sclerosis, Sjogren's disease, type I diabetes, Hashimoto's disease, Guillain-Barre, autoimmune hepatitis, Still's disease, stiff person syndrome, ulcerative colitis, and Crohn's disease, among others. Unfortunately for most people with **autoimmune disease**, it typically takes multiple years of living with symptoms before a diagnosis is made (Shomon, 2002) and the blood work starts to reflect the symptoms that the patient is reporting. During this time, people typically experience a feeling of being misunderstood, not taken seriously, doubting themselves, and are often told that they should seek out psychotherapy because they are likely somatizing something emotional, only to eventually end up in their doctor's office or hospital with organ failure and or some other medical crisis.

Being a psychoanalytically oriented clinical psychologist, I was quick to think about the meanings of my symptoms when I experienced my first lupus flare. A flare occurs when one's immune system is hyperactivated and attacks a part or parts of a person's body, causing significant inflammation which results in especially unpleasant and disruptive symptoms. As an intern in my last year of graduate school, working many intense hours with hospitalized patients diagnosed with medical illness and spending sleepless nights attempting to complete my dissertation, I attributed the swelling of my joints, exhaustion, hair loss, brain fog, and multiple rashes on my body as solely a reaction to stress. I did to myself what many people with **autoimmune disease** often experience others doing to them—I dismissed the very serious medical components of my symptoms. I was barely 30 years old after all, attended yoga four times a week, and never thought about my health. I was extremely lucky that one of my supervisors, a psychiatrist, insisted that I see a primary care physician because of these symptoms, and I found myself in the very privileged position of receiving a diagnosis and medical treatment immediately after the initial blood work, which is quite rare.

Thinking back on my life after receiving that diagnosis, I did recognize that I had bizarre symptoms throughout my twenties that didn't seem serious enough to address and that I didn't recognize were related to each other. I wonder if I had sought medical attention earlier, perhaps my experience would have been more consistent with the average six-year time frame to diagnosis (Lupus Foundation of America, 2024). More in line with the typical trajectory of living with an **autoimmune disease**, 13 years after being diagnosed with lupus, I was also diagnosed with rheumatoid arthritis and early Sjogren's disease.

It has been an interesting journey sitting both in the position of the patient with the **autoimmune disease** and of the psychologist with an **autoimmune disease**. Since my last year of internship and throughout my career post graduate school, I have worked with patients who have been diagnosed with various **autoimmune diseases**. Not all my patients know that I have **autoimmune diseases**, but something that I find interesting is that all of them have sought me out because they know I have experience working with this population, have written for various organizations that support these populations, or because I am involved with specific foundations that provide resources and raise funds to help these populations. What I have learned is that feeling understood is something that most people hope for when seeking out therapy, but for people with **autoimmune disease** it can often feel like extensive knowledge of what it is like to live with **autoimmune disease** is a prerequisite for their choice of therapist. Most folks who have an **autoimmune disease** repeatedly experience having their reality invalidated. This adds a layer of worry to the process of seeking out a therapist. "This is one of the biggest psychological tormentors of the invisibly ill: the disconnect between the way you feel and the constant refrain from family and friends that you look just fine" (Ramey, 2020, p. 37). Often reluctant to seek out therapy to begin with because they have likely been told that their symptoms are "all in their head" or that they "look fine," the idea of having their experience invalidated once again, by a therapist, can feel terrifying.

Receiving an autoimmune diagnosis can be traumatic for a number of reasons, which will be discussed in the following chapter. Not being aware of how to engage with people who have **autoimmune disease** in therapy may not only be unhelpful but may also cause harm. Mental health professionals who want to work with patients who live with **autoimmune disease** must first and foremost educate themselves about these diseases and how they can drastically impact a person's life over time, from pre-diagnosis, to diagnosis, and post-diagnosis. This book provides some basic yet important information about some of the common experiences, struggles, and fears of people living with **autoimmune disease**. Potential pitfalls are identified and recommendations for how to help patients make meaning of their illness are given. My hope is that this book serves as a useful guide to mental health professionals working with this population and that it is just the first of many resources to come specifically for working with **autoimmune disease** populations.

2

THE ROLE OF TRAUMA:
PRE-DIAGNOSIS AND BEYOND

S EVERAL YEARS AGO, I attended a networking event for mental
health professionals where I found myself engaged in a conversation
with two other psychologists who I was meeting for the first time. One
of the women asked, "What is your specialty?" I told her that I specialize
in working with people who have invisible medical illnesses, primarily
autoimmune and gynecological diseases. "Oh. **Autoimmune disease**.
Isn't that pretty much a reaction to unprocessed trauma?" she asked.
"Well, no. Sometimes that could be a part of it, but it is so much more
complicated. Sometimes being diagnosed and living with illness is the
trauma," I replied. Even though this was not the first time that I had
had this conversation with other professionals in the field, I remember
feeling frustrated with this conversation and with the lack of education
and awareness of mental health professionals when it came to **autoimmune diseases**.

THE UNKNOWN

Some of the misconceptions about the role of trauma and unprocessed
emotions in **autoimmune diseases** stem from an inability to sit with the
unknown. I have frequently encountered discourse around **autoimmune
diseases** specifically around fibromyalgia and myalgic encephalomyelitis

7

(previously known as "chronic fatigue syndrome") that pathologizes those who suffer from them as having unprocessed trauma, repressed emotions, or problematic thoughts and behaviors. The fact that an agreed upon etiology of these illnesses is unknown makes it easier for mental health professionals to speculate and endorse unsupported descriptions of what causes and how we can treat **autoimmune diseases**.

For example, in the introduction of his book *The Divided Mind* (2006), Dr. John Sarno includes fibromyalgia as one of the many "psychosomatic" ailments that people suffer from and asserts that these seemingly physical disorders have their origins in unconscious emotions. He continues to liken these psychosomatic symptoms as akin to the "hysterical" symptoms that Freud had treated and contends that the way in which unprocessed and unconscious emotions will present are determined by what is in "vogue." "Hysterical signs and symptoms are out of fashion" (Sarno, 2006, p. 43). Sarno then goes on to say that what "is in" is "low back pain, 'sciatica,' neck and shoulder pain, 'fibromyalgia,' 'carpal tunnel syndrome,' knee pain, hip pain, … and gastrointestinal symptoms" (2006, p43). He recommends psychodynamic psychotherapy to help patients identify and express their repressed emotions, which he asserts will also help them physically feel better.

Cognitive-behavioral researchers have also perpetuated the myth that these specific autoimmune illnesses (i.e. fibromyalgia and ME) are "all in the patient's mind." For example, Wessely and colleagues (1989, 1991) and Vercoulen et al. (1998) assert that certain cognitions and behaviors perpetuate the fatigue and impairment of those with ME. The Dysfunctional Belief Theory, one such cognitive-behavioral theory, assumes that there is no underlying medical pathology causing the symptoms and that patients are being hypervigilant to normal bodily sensations as a result of disrupted sleep, stress, and sedentary behavior (Wessely et al., 1989, 1991). However, consistent with what most patients and patient organizations assert, other empirical findings suggest that this cognitive-behavioral model is not accurate for this population and does not lead to symptom relief (Song & Jason, 2005; Sunnquist, 2016; Wilshire et al. 2017).

There is very little research on other **autoimmune diseases** apart from fibromyalgia and ME. One study (Bookwalter et al., 2020) looked at the relationship between PTSD and **autoimmune disease**, specifically rheumatoid arthritis, systemic lupus, multiple sclerosis, and inflammatory bowel disease in military personnel. They followed the participants for five years and found that those who were diagnosed with PTSD were at higher risk (58 percent) of developing one of these **autoimmune diseases**. Behavioral factors such as smoking, drinking, and BMI did not impact on the results, and results did not significantly differ based on combat experience or childhood physical or sexual trauma. The significant factor was the PTSD diagnosis itself, supporting that there is some relationship between trauma and the development of **autoimmune diseases**. Bookwalter and colleagues (2020) assert that their findings suggest that **autoimmune disease** may in part occur due to the biological changes that take place in the bodies of those with PTSD, which may adversely affect the immune system through increased inflammatory activity, changes in immune-related gene expression, and accelerated senescence of immune cells.

As indicated by the Bookwalter et al. 2020 study, a subset of **autoimmune disease** patients may indeed have a history of trauma, and as supported by what we see in our practices, they may also have unprocessed traumas, unconscious difficult emotions, or severely maladaptive cognitions and behaviors. However, many do not. In my own practice, I have seen patients with **autoimmune disease** who aside from their disease are the pinnacle of mental and physical health. These patients eat well, exercise, manage their daily stress with meditation and yoga, take natural supplements, and are active in processing difficult experiences in therapy, and yet continue to end up very physically ill and at times are medically hospitalized. There is still so much we do not understand about the role of genetics, the body, and the interaction between the body and lived experiences. Further, although psychotherapy can significantly help a patient cope with their illness, increase treatment adherence, and even assist in improving the patient's quality of life, there is no empirical evidence that psychotherapy will result in significant changes in **autoimmune disease** activity itself. For example, Conceicao, et al., 2019, found that psychoanalytic psychotherapy improves coping, depression and anxiety in patients with lupus, as well as improved medication adherence, but does not create any significant change in disease activity scores. Similarly, Navarrete-Navarrete et al., (2010) found that cognitive-behavioral therapy also improved quality of life, depression, and anxiety in patients with lupus, but did not affect disease activity or result in immunological changes.

WHAT WE DO KNOW

What we know is that stress increases inflammation, in which case trauma, difficult unprocessed emotions, or the ways in which one thinks about things certainly can play a role in the development of an **autoimmune disease**, but it is apparent that this is not the full story. We also know that **autoimmune diseases** have a genetic predisposition and that not everyone with this predisposition will develop the disease. Why is that? Unknown. However, we do know that "widespread inflammation and multisystemic neuropathology" is a piece of what results in ME (Carruthers et al., 2011, p. 327) and in many **autoimmune diseases** in general. Psychotherapy can at times be very helpful in mitigating the extent of the inflammatory process in **autoimmune disease**, by helping patients to better manage their stress and work through difficult emotions and/or trauma. However, we must be very careful to acknowledge that this does not mean that **autoimmune diseases** are not real medical disorders that require ongoing medical attention, and we must not confuse the benefits of psychotherapy with a cure for the disease itself. This may seem like an obvious statement to some; however, unfortunately I have too often encountered mental health providers who have talked about patients with **autoimmune disease** as if their physical symptoms were solely the product of behavioral, cognitive, and emotional factors with a complete negation of the genetic and biological realities.

AUTOIMMUNE DISEASE: SERIOUS ILLNESS OR AFTERTHOUGHT?

Reflective of the multiple ways in which **autoimmune diseases** live in the spaces of the unknown and of the invisible, is the following: In the very thoroughly edited book, *Health Psychology, 5th Edition* (Marks, Murray, & Estacio, 2018), there are entire chapters written about cardiac patients, cancer patients, and AIDS and HIV patients. There are no chapters on **autoimmune diseases** but there is a catch-all chapter on chronic illness where several illnesses, not specifically autoimmune, are lumped together.

One of these illnesses is myalgic encephalomyelitis (ME). The section discusses physicians' historical frustration with these patients because there is no one known etiology and no one known treatment (Marks, Murray, & Estacio, 2018). The dearth of information in *Health Psychology* parallels the reality of how these medical conditions are treated as after thoughts as opposed to very serious, life-changing, and at times life-threatening conditions. ME and fibromyalgia are not the only **autoimmune diseases** nor the most life-threatening, despite being the only diseases primarily attended to in the literature. For example, multiple sclerosis, type I diabetes, and lupus can be extremely serious and life threatening. Rheumatoid arthritis, ulcerative colitis, Crohn's disease, and Still's disease, like ME and fibromyalgia, can severely impact a person's quality of life. Why aren't we writing about or researching these conditions? Have we created a narrative where **autoimmune diseases** only refer to two out of the many types of **autoimmune diseases**? Have we already decided as a field that there is nothing more to understand about this body of illness?

WORD TO THE WISE

When meeting a patient for the first time, never lead with the suggestion that working through unprocessed trauma, repressed emotions, or maladaptive cognitions and behaviors will help with their physical autoimmune symptoms. This is the fastest route to ending a treatment before it has begun. Likely, the only thing the patient will hear is, "It is your fault that you are sick," or, "It is all in your mind." There is no rush. Exploration of stress, trauma, and difficult emotions will inevitably emerge as a byproduct of the patient living with the **autoimmune disease**. There is already so much happening to the patient and their body that is not in their control. Let them have some control over where they take the therapy.

It is important to consider how we as mental health professionals, much like medical doctors, similarly enact the invisibility and the dismissing of our patients with **autoimmune diseases** when we limit our understanding of them because it is too difficult to tolerate the unknown. When we assume that our patient's **autoimmune disease** stems solely from psychological factors, we may actually be repeating the trauma of patients having been invalidated and dismissed repeatedly by their medical providers and others.

The key is not to assume that trauma, depression, anxiety, or stress predates the onset of autoimmune symptoms, even if they may. Let the patient begin with their story, and you will likely hear about the trauma experienced while trying to identify a diagnosis, the trauma experienced when their body failed and continues to fail them in a profound way, the trauma experienced when someone else with the same diagnosis dies, the trauma experienced due to persistent microaggressions around medical illness and/or disability. They will have plenty of trauma and emotionally laden stories to tell that come with living with an **autoimmune disease**, and that is very likely where the patient would like to start. So, sit with the unknown and listen.

MEDICAL TRAUMA

It is ironic how many patients with **autoimmune diseases** go to doctors for help and oftentimes receive more pain, not only because they may not be taken seriously but also because they often endure repeated invasive and at times painful procedures. Some of these experiences can at times even be traumatic for the patients. Many people who live with **autoimmune diseases** often speak about the medical traumas that they experience.

Mariana, a woman with an **autoimmune disease** that caused her excruciating pain in her abdominal area, went to the emergency room as an adolescent and was told that she must be pregnant and hiding it from her parents. This woman had never had sex and repeated several times to the doctor that it was not possible that she was pregnant. She was sent home without care. It took almost a decade for her to be properly diagnosed as a result of not having been taken seriously or provided with adequate treatment. Once receiving the correct diagnosis, she required multiple surgeries as part of the correct treatment regimen which brought her the relief that she could have had years ago.

Another woman, Monique, was told that her chest pressure and persistent cough would subside if she simply exercised more and went to psychotherapy to manage her stress. Monique had already been in therapy for many years and exercised regularly. After continuously being dismissed by her doctor, she insisted that he order scans to assess why she was having these symptoms, which determined that she had pericarditis, inflammation of the lining around the heart. After finding a new doctor, she was prescribed the appropriate medication and finally received an autoimmune diagnosis. These examples are quite representative of what people, mostly women, endure while on their search for medical help. Some patients have even told me that they deliberately do not wear makeup to their medical appointments, hoping that if they do not look well, they will be taken more seriously.

After experiencing unbearable pelvic pain for weeks, Gina had to endure a series of gynecological tests and biopsies that were so painful that ever since, the idea of visiting a gynecologist throws her into a panic. Many of these tests, the biopsies, and the repeated vulnerability of being undressed or wearing just a gown while a doctor looks at you with doubt can be experienced by some patients as extremely invasive and even violating. Do not dismiss these patients' accounts of these experiences as dramatic or exaggerated! The fear and vulnerability of these medical interactions can be just as terrifying as a car accident, a violent assault, or a sexual transgression.

Another large piece of the medical trauma that many patients with **autoimmune diseases** experience is the fear of the "what may come." For example, many patients who have been diagnosed with an **auto-immune disease** are afraid of calling their doctor when they are not feeling well because they worry that it will be recommended that they have more tests done or that they will need another scan or additional medications. The fear here is twofold. On the one hand, the tests and/ or scans themselves can be triggering of previous trauma around tests and scans, and on the other hand, there is the fear that more disturbing information will come from these tests or scans.

For example, Anya was feeling very stiff in her hip and knee joints, and for weeks avoided telling her doctor because of her fear about what would be found. She waited in hopes that she would feel better with time and not need a medical appointment. She eventually called her doctor when her symptoms did not subside, and her doctor ordered an MRI of her pelvic area. The idea of yet another MRI was triggering of Anya's previous scan, which had resulted in unpleasant results, and she was extremely anxious heading into this MRI appointment. Following the MRI, the results indicated that she had an abnormal sacral-iliac joint that was contributing to her stiffness and pain, yet there was nothing she could do to reverse this abnormality. This is the fear of the "what may come" when visiting physicians-- the fear of what frightening news will come next.

There is so much unpredictability around **autoimmune diseases** with respect to course, prognosis, and development of additional autoimmune diagnoses. Simply having an autoimmune diagnosis can elicit the fears of "what may come." As a patient you hear from your doctors all of the possibilities that may or may never come to fruition, but which are never forgotten. For example, you might be told that you may exhibit neurological or cognitive disturbances. You could be told that you may not be able to carry a fetus to term. You are told that having this diagnosis makes it more likely that you will develop others. You may hear that you could have organ damage. The "what may come" is likely lurking in the background more often than not, and what to a person without an **autoimmune disease** may seem benign, could be terrifying to a person who has an **autoimmune disease**. For example, you may find a patient's obsession with a small rash a bit odd, yet to the person with the **autoimmune disease** the rash may feel like a signal of a flare to come.

WORD TO THE WISE

Try not to act on your impulse to help. It can be tempting to offer a bit of advice or a seemingly helpful piece of information; however, it is best to assume that the patient already knows what you are about to tell them and that you are not the first to offer it to them. For example, being told to try putting hydrocortisone on the aforementioned rash will not bring any comfort at all. The patient needs to have the fear of the "what may come" recognized by you. The goal for you as the clinician is to hear the patient out and to tolerate sitting with their fears of "what may come" in order to help the patient feel recognized and understood. Only then, after you have allowed sufficient space for the patient's fears, can you begin to brainstorm a plan together for how the patient may come to feel more empowered to address their symptoms and their fears in the way that feels most helpful to them. This process will allow for the patient to feel contained and understood.

A qualitative study conducted by Pothemont and colleagues (2021) examined patients' perspectives on medical trauma. The participants in the study had a diagnosis of inflammatory bowel disease (IBD), which includes Crohn's disease and ulcerative colitis, and they were also assessed for post-traumatic stress symptoms using the Post-Traumatic Stress Disorder Symptom Scale for DSM5 (PSSI-5). A semi-structured interview was then conducted to identify which aspects of living with IBD were particularly scary or traumatic. Participants who met criteria for PTSD, cited hospitalization and/or surgery as a source of trauma.

Five main themes emerged from the interview data. The themes were uncertainty about IBD, information exchange and quality, procedures, surgeries, and coping strategies.

More specifically, the uncertain nature of when IBD symptoms would occur and how severe they would be, were especially upsetting to patients. For some patients, severe symptoms would result in anxiety or panic attacks, as did hospitalization or surgery. Not having control over one's body was also reported as very distressing. Feeling knowledgeable about all treatment options was found to be a protective factor against post-traumatic stress symptoms. However, uncertainty around new treatments and their side effects created anxiety, and medications such as steroids and immunosuppressants which are frequently used for treatment of most **autoimmune diseases** came with additional concerns. In particular, patients felt frightened by the uncontrollable mood changes that came with high doses of steroids, such as anger and anxiety, as well as bodily changes not in their control like weight gain and excessive sweating. Immunosuppressants were of concern because of the unpredictable side effects and potential for infection.

Pothemont and colleagues (2021) additionally found that patients reported that insensitive and hasty or rushed communication by doctors also contributed to their experience of feeling traumatized by the medical world. This negative experience for patients oftentimes resulted in patients looking up information on the internet, which often left patients fearful about what was happening to them, especially during hospitalization. Trauma was also reported in relation to the way doctors communicated to patients about surgical procedures and subsequently around scars left on the patient's body post-surgery.

It is critical to hold in mind how our patients may experience trauma throughout various moments of seeking medical attention and care. There is the trauma that may come from all of the procedures and interactions just explored, and as will be discussed, there is the trauma that comes with receiving a chronic and in some instances potentially life-threatening diagnosis. Additionally, for many people who live with **autoimmune disease**, there will also be the trauma that comes from persistent microaggressions due to gender and/or racial bias.

DIAGNOSIS

It may be easy to assume that patients would be happy to receive a diagnosis after living through years of trying to be heard and taken seriously when expressing their symptoms. It is not that simple. Patients typically have ambivalent feelings about receiving a diagnosis. There is a great sense of relief in finally having a name for what they have been experiencing for so many years. It can feel like it legitimizes them in the medical world, to their friends, their family, and their employers. However, receiving a chronic and at times life-threatening diagnosis is a terrifying and possibly traumatic moment in a person's life.

I recall the moment I was told that I had lupus, and I remember thinking to myself, "What the hell is lupus?" I had never heard of lupus before and the only words from my doctor that I could hold onto were "chronic illness," "no cure," "medication for life," "may affect your ability to have a healthy pregnancy," and "can affect any organ." Who wants to live with all that? Although it is helpful to know that you are not "making the symptoms up," most people would feel equally legitimized or satisfied with a less life-altering diagnosis, such as being told they have an infection that can be cured with antibiotics or having a virus that will pass on its own time. An autoimmune diagnosis is a forever changed diagnosis. I was crushed when I was told that I could no longer spend time in the sun and that in fact I would have to cover up my skin in the sun to prevent the increased potential for a flare and painful rashes. It was an extreme loss for a person like me who adores the outdoors and the beach especially.

Autoimmune disease is a diagnosis that can have different implications over time. It can be mild now and become more severe in time, or not. In some cases, it can put a person at higher risk for certain cancers. It may not be affecting your heart or brain currently yet may (or may not) do so in the future…and the scariest part is that there is no way to know. Receiving an autoimmune diagnosis is the beginning of how the fear of the "what may come" develops. Diagnosis can also be the start of meaning making. It is extremely difficult to make meaning out of one's illness when that illness has no name, no treatment, and frequently no acknowledgement by others. I am not saying that it is impossible to make meaning out of the difficult situation of being ill with a condition that has no name; however, it is very challenging.

Most people who live with **autoimmune disease** are able to start making meaning of their illness after they have been diagnosed and can begin to have a framework for what is happening to them. They can now know what kind of medical specialists to see, they now have access to a language that they can use to communicate with doctors, family, and friends about what they are experiencing in their bodies. They have access to support groups, a community of others with the same diagnosis, and information about what to possibly expect from said illness. Because they now have this framework, one can start to make peace with what it means to live with their specific illness, even if their diagnosis is an unspecified **autoimmune disease**. How the process of meaning making unfolds will be discussed in detail in Chapter 7.

INTERSECTIONALITY OF TIME & MULTIPLE TRAUMAS

Time and age intersect with the trauma of living with an **autoimmune disease** in a way that creates ripples from the past through the present and into the future. Traumas from the past may resurface while the patient may also simultaneously be trying to process the potential trauma of diagnosis, and of holding the fear of the "what may come." When a patient reaches out because they want help with coping with their **autoimmune disease**, one of the first things that I always tell them is that being diagnosed and living with an **autoimmune disease** can be traumatic, and that when something traumatic happens, it can resurface unresolved traumas from the past. One patient, Gabrielle, expressed immense relief when I shared this with her and she immediately went on to tell me that since she received her MS diagnosis, trauma around her relationship with her mother felt very present, especially since becoming ill necessitated her to accept help from her mother who she would have otherwise kept at more of a distance.

I have already discussed how the time period involving diagnosis itself can be traumatic, as well as the trauma that can come from the medical world itself, and the trauma that stems from repetitive invalidation of the patient's experience. Beyond diagnosis, there are additional traumas that can emerge as a result of daily experiences that come with living with an **autoimmune disease**. For example, getting a cold or the flu, which for people who do not have **autoimmune disease** is just getting a cold or the flu.

However, for those living with an **autoimmune disease**, it can come with a flare, a hospital visit, or significant complications. If a person has had one of these experiences following getting a common cold, they may now experience tremendous anxiety around getting sick and or exhibit other symptoms of trauma when they are close to an obviously sick person or when they themselves get sick again. Other daily experiences that can also contribute to the triggering of trauma symptoms is learning about another person dying who was diagnosed with same condition, having a poor reaction to a medication, having medication cause other significant health problems, being chastised for taking a seat on a crowded subway because you do not "look like" you need it, not being able to engage in sexual activity, pregnancy loss due to the illness and/or medications, difficulty finding and/or sustaining a romantic relationship because of your medical needs, and the multiple losses that come with illness that will be discussed in Chapter 3.

The age at which the person is diagnosed and/or suffering from symptoms can also contribute to additional traumas. For example, most people with type I diabetes are diagnosed in childhood and adolescence, as opposed to most people with lupus who are diagnosed typically between 20–40 years old, which is also different from people with Guillain-Barre where the age of diagnosis is most commonly over 50. It is crucial that mental health professionals consider the ways in which being diagnosed with an illness at a particular age comes with specific losses and potential traumas.

For example, imagine being an adolescent who is diagnosed with type I diabetes and needs to wear a glucose monitor and/or inject oneself with insulin. This adolescent may experience fear of their peers finding out about their illness or bullying them because of it. These fears would not be irrational given how adolescent insecurities often drive adolescents to prey on those with vulnerabilities. This teen may very likely be experiencing bullying. The fears or even feelings of shame at times may hinder this adolescent's openness to romantic relationships or sexual exploration. This adolescent may not be able to participate in group sports or teams depending on how much their health is affected. They may feel very alone.

Other **autoimmune diseases** that are diagnosed in women of childbearing age, such as lupus and endometriosis[1] can come with a very different set of potential traumas and/or losses. Pregnancy can be difficult for people who live with both of these **autoimmune diseases**. Endometriosis, which causes tissue that should normally grow inside of the uterus to grow on the outside of the uterus, can cause serious problems with fertility. Many women with endometriosis are unable to naturally conceive. They also experience tremendous pain as a result of tissue growing in places where it is not meant to grow. Sexual intercourse is extremely painful for women who have endometriosis and oftentimes is not possible at all without significant physical therapy. Women who live with lupus are at increased risk for miscarriage and are at increased risk for flares throughout pregnancy and after childbirth. Most rheumatologists recommend that a woman who has lupus be symptom-free for at least six months before attempting to conceive. Additionally, pregnancy can come with complications for women with lupus, such as high blood pressure, kidney disease, and preeclampsia.

There are some **autoimmune diseases** such as Guillain-Barre that tend to present in people over 50, although not always; however, the vast majority of **autoimmune diseases** present during younger ages where people typically do not think about loss of bodily control, disability, the human body's fragility, or mortality. People who live with **autoimmune disease** break through a denial of death that the majority of non-medically ill people under 50 walk around with every day. This denial is shattered when your joints fail you or when you struggle to find words

---

[1] Currently there is debate over whether Endometriosis is an **autoimmune disease**; however, it is established that there is a significant relationship between Endometriosis and other **autoimmune diseases** (Shigesi et al, 2019) and Endometriosis is often included on lists of other **autoimmune diseases** (e.g. Global Autoimmune Institute, 2024).

that you know that you know. This denial breaks when you go into kidney failure or when you wake up one day and cannot walk.

People in their childhood, twenties, thirties, and even forties usually do not acknowledge the realities of the body's fragility or of mortality. These things are commonly relegated to the elderly. Having this denial of death shattered can definitely be traumatic, at least in a society like the one in the United States where discussion about the inevitability and natural order of death is not something that is encouraged but rather is heard in whispers or is completely avoided. It is quite terrifying when you are at the prime of your life and suddenly your body fails you. Suddenly you start to wonder whether you will be able to work, have a relationship, live to have children, or live to see your children grow.

INTERSECTIONALITY OF RACE, SEX AND PRIVILEGE WITH INVISIBILITY AND MICRO-AGGRESSIVE TRAUMA

Miranda is an African American woman in her late twenties who was diagnosed with lupus as a child. During a particularly painful flare, she went to the emergency room for care and instead was met with hostility and suspicion. Miranda shared that her pain was not taken seriously and after waiting for hours was told to leave because it was "suspected that she was seeking pain meds." Miranda was extremely hurt by this experience and subsequently felt hopeless and alone. Unfortunately, this is not the first time Miranda had this experience when going to the hospital for help. Miranda told me that as a black woman she has had many experiences with health care providers who did not take her symptoms seriously and we discussed the role of implicit bias in these interactions. As Miranda told me about her experiences, I thought about my own experiences as a white woman who although has felt unheard and invalidated by healthcare providers, has never been accused of "medication seeking."

According to the NIH, about 85 percent of people who are diagnosed with an **autoimmune disease** are women and for some **autoimmune diseases** (e.g. autoimmune hepatitis, lupus, scleroderma), people of color are disproportionately affected (Lee et al, 2018; NIH). The reasons for these gender-based differences are not fully understood, yet sex hormones, in particular estrogen, are thought to play a significant role in the development of these illnesses (NIH). Another theory is that microchimerism that occurs during pregnancy plays a role in the development of **autoimmune disease** (Shrivastava et al, 2019). Microchimerism occurs when genetically distinct cells are found in a person's body, meaning that they are not the person's own cells but rather cells that came from another person's body. This was initially discovered when male cells were found in women's bodies and understood as coming from these women's fetuses during gestation. However, microchimerism can also occur from twin to twin in utero, through blood transfusion and organ transplant, and therefore is something that can occur in males and intersex people as well (Nelson, 2002). Additionally, studies on various **autoimmune diseases** have both lent support and cast doubt on the role of microchimerism in relation to these diseases (Nelson, 2002; Shrivastava et al, 2019).

As previously mentioned, in addition to gender disparities, there are also racial disparities among those who have certain **autoimmune diseases**. For example, one study that used a large national electronic medical record database of over 52 million people found that multiracial **autoimmune disease** rates were significantly higher than Caucasian rates in almost all of the 22 **autoimmune diseases** that were included in the study (Roberts & Erdei, 2019). However, according to the NIH, the epidemiological evidence to support higher prevalence of these diseases in certain racial groups is complicated. For example, there are significant environmental influences that contribute to the onset of these diseases, including diet, infectious agents, occupational and residential exposures, and stress. The disparities found between races may not necessarily be indicative of a biological difference and rather may be a factor of higher exposure to these environmental influences that people of color may be exposed to with more frequency and consistency than Caucasians. Again, this is complicated because there are some **autoimmune diseases** where there do not seem to be any racial disparities. There is still a lot to learn.

What we do know is that both women and especially women of color are often dismissed by healthcare providers in multiple ways in general. Phrases that are often heard about women who are expressing a medical concern are, "You are being dramatic;" "You are exaggerating;" "They are just seeking attention;" "You are fragile and weak;" or, in the case of women of color, "They are medication seeking." Women are treated for pain less aggressively than men (Hoffmann & Tarzian, 2001) and are more likely than men to be told that their pain is psychosomatic (National Pain Report, 2016). Women of color are likely to experience both gender and racial implicit bias. Implicit racial bias can result in poor patient assessment, less serious diagnoses, less effective treatment recommendations, poor pain management, fewer referrals to specialists, and less patient engagement (Rose, 2020). These microaggressions are destructive and over time can build up and result in yet another form of trauma.

I find it impossible to not question whether the lack of funding for autoimmune research is somehow not connected to who these diseases primarily impact—women and in some cases mostly women of color. In fact, according to the NIH, **autoimmune diseases** are a leading cause of death among young and middle aged women. The NIH spends roughly 44.7 billion dollars a year for research; however, spending on **autoimmune disease** has remained at only 2.6 percent of overall NIH obligations between 2013 through 2020, in contrast to increases seen in other NIH obligations during the same period (Autoimmune Association, 2024). This has obvious implications for advances in the treatment of these diseases. However, since long Covid has affected millions of people of all genders, races, and socioeconomic status worldwide, attention has been turned to studying the autoimmune-like symptoms found in long Covid, which will also benefit people who are living with **autoimmune diseases**. In fact, some very recent research (e.g. Chang et al., 2023; Sharma & Bayry, 2023) suggests that there could be an increased risk of **autoimmune disease** following Covid-19 infection, and among those who already have an **autoimmune disease**, there is evidence that a Covid-19 infection increases their risk of developing another **autoimmune disease** by 23 percent (Tesch et al, 2023). It is interesting to note that between 2020 and 2023, the years of the Covid-19 pandemic, global autoimmune disorder spending for treatments increased by $41 billion US dollars—almost double the increase between the years 2016 through 2019 (Mikulic, 2023).

There is a growing number of people who are diagnosed with and need treatment for **autoimmune diseases** (Miller, 2023) and whether or not this is due to Covid-19 is unknown. Nevertheless, Covid-19 has brought attention to **autoimmune diseases** like never before and this is a complicated matter for our patients. Although on the one hand patients may feel excited about the growing awareness of **autoimmune diseases**, which have historically been invisible in mainstream society and media, patients may also feel angry that their illness is only now garnering attention when people in power, people with privilege, and men are at increased risk for developing autoimmune-like symptoms following a Covid-19 infection. These diseases did not have to be ignored for so long.

WHEN WOMEN'S SUFFERING IS DISMISSED

In her co-authored book, *If You Have to Wear an Ugly Dress, Learn to Accessorize*, Karen Kemper, MSPH, PhD writes about her first doctor's appointment when she began to have symptoms of what was eventually diagnosed as Scleroderma, an **autoimmune disease**. She went to see her primary care physician and told him about the swelling in her hands and feet. Her feet were so swollen that she needed to buy larger shoes and her fingers so swollen that she had trouble using her hands. Her doctor told her that, "They would probably never know why her hands were swollen. And besides, this is really just a vanity problem" (McNamara & Kemper, 2011, p.10). Karen describes how she almost lost her finger to the disease as a result of this doctor's dismissive attitude.

Unfortunately, Karen's story is not unique. The medical field has not always treated women kindly and we know that there is ample gender bias. The world of mental health is not so different. Reflecting on how mental health professionals have historically treated women, it is easy to understand how Sarno could compare fibromyalgia to Freud's hysterical patients, patients who exhibited unexplained physical symptoms such as paralysis. Although Freud's original theory, the seduction theory, posited that most of his patients experienced sexual abuse as children (Freud, 1896), he abandoned this theory only one year later and created his theory of the psychosexual stages of development.

There are many hypotheses for why he chose to abandon his original theory. One reason is that Freud experienced disapproval from his peers and was pressured to revise the theory (Masson, 1984). This was a time period where childhood sexual abuse, or sexual abuse of any nature was not acknowledged as a phenomenon that occurred with as much frequency as we now know that it does. As such, Freud's theory evolved from considering that abuse actually occurred, to conceptualizing that the patient had a fantasy of having sex with their opposite sex parent. Thus, the blame moves from the perpetrator to the victim, who in the cases of hysteria were usually female, and in effect dismisses their trauma.

Blame for ailments were easily placed on women throughout the history of mental health, including blaming mothers for their child's autism or schizophrenia. Given this history, it would not be surprising to make the leap that female patients with **autoimmune diseases** would be blamed for their illness. I recall a conversation with a colleague many years ago who struggled in their work with a patient who had an **autoimmune disease**. My colleague was struggling with frustration around how frequently their patient was ill and needed to reschedule appointments. They didn't know how to handle this situation, so I simply asked them, "How would you handle this if she were a cancer patient?" This one question cleared up so much for my colleague. Immediately they were able to connect to how they would approach the situation if their patient had cancer. This is the type of bias that comes with **autoimmune diseases**, and in my belief, stems primarily from the reality that it is mostly a women's illness.

It was difficult for my colleague to take their patient's illness and symptoms seriously, and their impulse was to understand the **autoimmune disease** as a conversion disorder or a psychosomatic phenomenon, which dismisses so much of the patient's reality and the reality of actual medical components and complications. In conversion disorder, there are physical symptoms that are outside of the patient's voluntary control, yet no underlying neurological or medical disease. The physical symptoms seen in conversion disorder are understood as masking underlying emotional distress. Conversion disorder is extremely rare, with only two to five cases out of 100,000 per year. The incidence of **autoimmune diseases** is not well documented, but the prevalence is about 10 million people in the United States alone (Johns Hopkins, 2024).

People do not die from conversion disorder, but many people die from **autoimmune diseases** every year. As stated earlier, it is one of the leading causes of death in young adult and middle aged women (NIH). In fact, 30 years ago before there were treatments for lupus, the life expectancy was five years post diagnosis (McNamara & Kemper, 2011). In conversion disorder, there is no underlying neurological or medical condition; however, people with **autoimmune diseases** often have multiple neurological and multi-systemic abnormalities. For example, part of diagnosing multiple sclerosis is using an MRI to look for lesions on their brain and spine. About a third of people who have systemic lupus will have lupus nephritis, also known as kidney disease (Madhok, 2015). In rheumatoid arthritis, inflammation of the joints is so bad that there is deformity in the fingers and toes. Diagnosing all **autoimmune diseases** partly involves abnormality in the results of blood work. As stated earlier, we also know that there is a genetic component to these diseases. There is clearly something very wrong medically when it comes to **autoimmune diseases**.

The mind and body interact in ways that we are just beginning to understand. Perhaps there is something medical underlying conversion disorder as well and we do not yet have the diagnostic tools to identify it. I am in no way attempting to minimize the suffering of those with conversion disorder. Rather, I want to highlight the ways in which suffering of women is historically quickly dismissed as unprocessed emotion, and in some cases it may very well be. However, when we as mental health providers comment on **autoimmune diseases** as "just conversion disorder," we are associating **autoimmune diseases** with unprocessed emotion and once again dismissing the very real physical danger and suffering that come from living with this category of illness, and focusing only on trying to figure out what emotions have not yet been processed will not help the patient cope with their hospital visits and/or pain.

Almost every year, I take part in a walk with the Lupus Foundation of America to raise money for lupus. I am always moved by the signs and T-shirts that many of the other walkers display. I have seen signs that say, "I walk in my mom's memory," "I walk for my wife," "I walk for my friend, R.I.P." **autoimmune diseases** are debilitating illnesses and, in some cases, can be life-threatening. A person who comes into therapy looking to talk about the suffering that their **autoimmune disease** causes will likely feel misunderstood if you immediately start wondering about which unprocessed emotions are the cause of their physical symptoms.

WORD TO THE WISE

Think about your own unconscious gender and racial biases. How may they be informing your understanding of your patient? Think about all the fears and stressors that your patient with an **autoimmune disease** is dealing with. Did they experience microaggressions from their doctor? How may you be microaggressing? Could your conceptualization of your patient be skewed because of your patient's gender or race? Think about all the comments you have heard from your peers about people who have your patient's diagnosis or about the diagnosis itself. How many of these comments have been derogatory or condescending? We are all capable of bias and microaggressions.

TRAUMA EVERYWHERE

There can be so much trauma involved when living with an **autoimmune disease**. As discussed, trauma can predate the diagnosis, it can occur during the time of diagnosis, and it often continues to occur after diagnosis and throughout the person's life. There are so many worries your patient may have related to loss. They may be concerned about losing their health insurance due to loss of work. They may be worried that they won't ever be able to work again. They could be worried about their relationships or their loved ones not understanding their physical pain. They may be afraid that they will die young. There could be so many traumas and fears present right now for you to help your patient to cope with. These potential fears and losses will now be discussed in Chapter 3. Strive to let your patients know that you can see all these fears and the realities of what it is like to live with an **autoimmune disease**. Start with that and you will see how powerful genuinely making an effort to understand your patient's struggle with their illness from their perspective can be.

3

LOSS, GRIEF, AND REPEAT...

THERE ARE PERIODS when I am doing well and feel healthy, and there are other times when I feel miserable. That is how **autoimmune diseases** typically present, with periods of ups and moments of down. Autoimmune flares come in and out of peoples' lives, with various frequencies and intensities from patient to patient, and even within the same patient. There is no rhyme or reason, just unpredictability—and, as discussed in Chapter 2, the patient's fear of "what may come" emerges from this. There are times when I feel healthy for very long periods, and I can catch myself believing that I am **autoimmune disease** free. These are also the moments in which I can find myself wondering if I just made it all up. I think to myself, "Maybe I was just being dramatic or was exaggerating how awful I felt, or maybe the blood work was wrong."

Watching myself write these words on paper, I recognize how sad it is that I could so easily erase my reality, the repeated blood taken over more than a decade of years, the repeated flares, and the pain. But I also know that there is a part of me that would love for my fantasy that I "made it all up" to be true because then I wouldn't have to suffer, live in fear of the "what may come," or experience the multiple losses that comes with living with an **autoimmune disease**. As I write, at this moment, I am experiencing a very unpleasant flare. The fantasy that I "made it all up" is immediately destroyed as my body erupts in rashes, swollen joints, pain, hair loss, ulcers throughout my body, fatigue, brain fog, swollen lymph nodes, nausea, dizziness, and disorientation. This is the moment when a patient who lives with **autoimmune disease** remembers, "Oh right. I *am* sick," and once again loses their hope for health. It is quite a painful loss.

Autoimmune diseases are at times compared to other illnesses that can be life threatening such as cancer and HIV. This is something that often upsets patients who live with **autoimmune diseases** and for good reason. For example, the phrase "at least it's not cancer" is something that patients who have **autoimmune disease** have heard all too often. These kinds of phrases imply that living with an **autoimmune disease** is not as terrible as living with cancer or HIV. Making comparisons between severe illnesses is horrendous in itself; however, it is also a false and inequivalent comparison. Most in the general population and perhaps many of us mental health professionals may equate certain illnesses like cancer and HIV with loss and grief, but what many people may not know is that the list of losses that can come with living with an **autoimmune disease** can feel infinite.

IMPACT ON QUALITY OF LIFE

Living with an **autoimmune disease** can have a tremendous impact on a person's quality of life. One study (Greenfield et al., 2017) compared quality of life scores of patients with systemic lupus, rheumatoid arthritis, systemic sclerosis, and idiopathic inflammatory myopathies to the average scores of the general population using the Short Form Health Survey Physical and Mental Component summary scores. They found that the quality-of-life scores for people diagnosed with any of these four **autoimmune diseases** were significantly lower than the average scores of the general population. The three **autoimmune disease** groups differed from each other; however, the group who scored closest to the general population, those with lupus, still scored more than one standard deviation below the general population. The participants diagnosed with the other three **autoimmune diseases** scored more than two standard deviations below the general population. These results suggest that there is a significant relationship between living with an **autoimmune disease** and a decreased quality of life.

Some research also suggests that treatments of **autoimmune diseases** impact patients' quality of life more than the disease itself (i.e. Behkar et al., 2022). A recent study (Behkar et al., 2022) investigated the quality of life of patients being treated for autoimmune bullous diseases. These are **autoimmune diseases** in which autoantibodies loosen molecular adhesions in the skin and mucosa, which results in blisters, erosions, and lesions. These skin conditions can be extremely painful and can be treated; however, as is the case for most **autoimmune diseases**, the treatments often come with significant side effects, which can also impact quality of life. The researchers assessed the patients' quality of life using the Treatment of Autoimmune Bullous Quality of Life Questionnaire (TABQOL). The results showed that there was a significant relationship between medication dose and TABQOL scores, suggesting the negative impact of these treatments on quality of life.

As mental health providers, we shouldn't just stop at the acknowledgment of "some impact on the quality of life" on our patients' lives. It is also important for us to understand and think about why quality of life is so greatly impacted by our patients' **autoimmune diseases** and their treatments. This is not because we can necessarily change the circumstances that influence our patients' quality of life, but so that our patients feel visible and recognized. As will be discussed, decreased quality of life in **autoimmune disease** patients, as likely with most chronic illnesses, is related to tremendous loss. There are multiple types of loss, some repeated, some one time, and some unbearable. Having a vivid picture of what these losses look like may not only help your patients but will also help you hold onto empathy when you may feel frustrated with your patients' complaints about their quality of life. It can help you stay connected to the reality that your patients may likely be in a process of continuous grief and mourning. The losses are…many.

THE LOSSES

Decreased quality of life for patients with **autoimmune disease** that either comes from the disease itself or from the treatments for the disease is often the product of multiple losses. The most obvious loss is the loss of health, both literally and with respect to the patient's own perception of themselves as a person without illness. As easy as it is to imagine that this would be a loss, it is not easy to accept when you are the one living with the disease. It is very difficult to grieve this loss when there isn't a finite loss of health but rather a roller coaster ride where the person flares up, feels very sick, and discovers that they have a chronic illness but then may have periods of remission and good health in between flares as well.

How does one make sense of this? A patient is tasked with coming to accept that they have this chronic diagnosis that will impact them for the rest of their life in some form and may go through a process of grieving the loss of their perception of health, only to find themselves feeling relatively healthy during other periods, while also wondering about awful things that may happen to them in the future. It is quite confusing. Each time a new period of flare emerges, the person goes through the experience of grief all over again, and as discussed in the previous chapter this can be traumatic, and hard for others who do not have an **autoimmune disease** to understand.

Infinite additional losses also come with the loss of health. For example, physically, a person who was a runner may no longer be able to run because their rheumatoid arthritis has affected their hips. Gina, a middle-aged woman who lives with lupus used to work long hours as a corporate attorney, but her fatigue became so severe that she needed to take a medical leave of absence and ultimately had to change her professional goals.

Personally, with the loss of my health came the loss of enjoying the sunshine. UVA and UVB light can trigger lupus flares, and unfortunately this is the case for me. During the summer months I must cover my body head to toe to protect myself from a flare, which isn't always successful. Simply walking in the sun for 10–15 minutes can result in painful and itchy rashes, fatigue, and terrible joint pain, so I cover up. It is a loss of a specific kind of carefreeness and spontaneity for me. Another woman, Cassandra, was a very active graduate student in her mid-twenties who was progressively feeling fatigued and weak but assumed it was because she was overworking herself. She woke up one day unable to walk and was diagnosed with multiple sclerosis. She had great difficulty walking for months before they found the correct medication for her. Carla, a woman living with lupus who desperately wanted to get pregnant, lost that possibility because she was too ill to take on the risk of pregnancy.

WORD TO THE WISE

These are just snippets of some patients' stories. It is important for their stories to be told, not to be unknown or invisible. It can be confusing for mental health professionals as well when witnessing patients who have **autoimmune diseases** fluctuate between feeling incredibly ill and feeling healthy. At times, it can even feel like you are speaking to two different people. If we as a field are not educated on the presentation of **autoimmune disease** patients with respect to how their health status can ebb and flow, and how these physical changes impact the patients' mood, frustration tolerance, energy, sense of hope, and interpersonal skills, then we may mistakenly perceive some of these patients as having certain mental health disorders that they do not. It is helpful to understand these different fluctuating parts of the patient, as just that—different fluctuating parts.

It is also useful to work with the patient to identify these different parts and have the patient give names to these parts. The names should be specific and have some meaning for the individual person. If both the patient and therapist can identify and name each particular state or part of the patient, then it is easier for the patient and therapist to hold in mind that these parts are only pieces of the patient and not the whole. Together, you can hold in mind that these states will not be permanently in the foreground but will come and go, and that parts beyond the pain and suffering of the patient continue to exist even if pain and suffering are the only parts front and center in the moment. This will be discussed more elaborately in Chapter 6.

REPEAT

After some time, some people who have **autoimmune diseases** may come to terms with loss of health and perhaps make some meaning out of it; however, people who live with **autoimmune diseases** are continuously grieving. The loss of health is not the only loss that comes with living with an **autoimmune disease** and there will be grief around a number of other losses. Perhaps one of the most difficult is the loss of life. It can be terrifying for someone living with an **autoimmune disease** to hear about someone who has the same diagnosis as them, having died. The loss can come in the form of knowing a person who died from the disease such as a family member (remember these diseases run in families), a member of a support group, or member of a foundation or organization. The loss can also be felt when hearing or reading about a celebrity who died from the disease. Following these experiences, our patients may find themselves not only grieving the life that was lost but also feeling grief around the possibility that they may lose their life in a similar way as well, which some patients will.

Tied to loss of health and fears of actual loss of life is the real possibility of loss of health insurance, loss of savings, and loss of health care. We all know how expensive health care can be with or without insurance coverage. Medical debt is a persistent problem in the United States and according to a Census Bureau analysis in 2019, 17 percent of U.S. households owed medical debt. Insurance premiums are high and out of pocket costs before meeting a deductible can be debilitating. Living with an **autoimmune disease** is expensive as there are frequent blood and urine analyses needed, MRIs, X-rays, physical therapies, complementary or alternative treatments that are recommended by doctors but not covered by insurance, and dieticians and other specialists, including mental health teams. These costs add up. Additionally, thanks to the Affordable Care Act, even though insurance companies cannot deny coverage due to pre-existing conditions, not all insurance options are regulated by the Affordable Care Act and insurance companies can still deny coverage or charge higher rates based on a patient's medical history (U.S. Department of Health & Human Services, 2024). In fact, this happened to me when I tried to obtain a new policy through a professional association. I was denied coverage when I applied for the plan that had a higher premium but lower deductible and broader coverage. I was told that due to my medical history, I would only be eligible for the cheaper plan with the high deductibles and limited coverage. How counterintuitive given that the people who need the care the most are the ones most often denied!

Many people who live with **autoimmune diseases** often rely on their jobs for both health insurance and income but are also often worried about their ability to continue working due to their illness. In many cases **autoimmune diseases** will be severe enough or progress to the point of inability to work. This will not be true for all patients with **autoimmune disease** and will depend on the specific disease, age of the patient, how far the disease has progressed, and the nature of the person's job. However, this does occur frequently enough that it is a common concern of patients who live with **autoimmune disease**. Sometimes patients need to take a temporary medical leave of absence and after a period of rest can return to work, and other times patients need to either go on disability or rely on a partner or family member for financial support.

There is so much loss and grief in these situations. Loss of livelihood, grief of a part of your professional identity, loss of colleagues and work friends, loss of feeling productive or generative, loss of a respected gaze from others, and as mentioned the loss of health insurance and income for medical expenses. Samantha is a married middle-aged mother of three who has had a very successful career in finance. After the birth of her second child, she became very ill and was subsequently diagnosed with scleroderma. Her condition was so severe that she needed to leave her job and rely on her partner to be the sole breadwinner of their family. Up until that time, Samantha was the primary breadwinner as her income was significantly more than her partner's. Not only was the financial strain a great loss, but she experienced a period of tremendous grief around her identity as a respected professional and perceived a loss of respect from her partner and peers. She lost her daily routine and structure as well as her experience of herself as a productive member of society. It took Samantha many months to grieve this loss before she could even begin to think about how she could still incorporate pieces of her professional identity into the framework that her life currently takes.

It is also important to note that although it is considered wrongful termination to cease a person's employment because of a medical condition or because they take a medical leave of absence, it may not be against the law in certain circumstances. Much like insurance companies have loopholes to deny coverage, an employer may terminate someone who is struggling due to a medical condition by claiming that a termination did not have to do with the illness, asserting that the employee did not meet the requirements of the job, and or claiming that the employee poses a direct threat to the health and safety of others in the workplace due to their disability (U.S. Department of Labor, 2025). People who live with **autoimmune disease** often carry this anxiety that they will be let go or seen as lazy or incompetent at their place of work because of the ways in which their illness may change the way they work compared to before they got ill. This anxiety accompanies a loss of trust in job security and at times loss of trust in the loyalty of an employer that historically was experienced as supportive.

Another repeated loss that people who live with **autoimmune disease** experience is the loss of hope for a cure. Although the medical community concurs that there are no cures for **autoimmune diseases** and only treatments to manage them, people who live with these diseases often hear about "miraculous cures" following various alternative treatments. These treatments can take the form of specific diets, use of supplements or herbs, acupuncture, various energy healing, and earthing. None of these treatments have been empirically supported as "cures" for **autoimmune diseases** but they can be helpful for some people with respect to managing their symptoms.

However, a well-meaning person living with an **autoimmune disease** may share with another **autoimmune disease** patient that they were "cured" by one of these treatments. The person who has just received this information may feel hope that this alternative treatment will cure their illness and they may also decide to try the treatment. In these situations, there is no way to really know what "cured" the person who initially tried the alternative treatment. There is also no way to know if the person was actually cured or if they were just in a flare-free period. We also know that the range of **autoimmune disease** presentation and symptoms are so wide that what works for one may not work for all. However, hearing that someone with the same or similar condition as you has been helped, makes it hard not to feel some hope that it could help you too. Unfortunately, oftentimes the treatment isn't the miracle cure that the patient was expecting, and the patient is left to grieve the loss of hope. There are so many alternative treatments to hear about and try and therefore this up and down of hope and loss of hope often occurs multiple times throughout the person's life while living with the illness.

The relationship a person has with their body is changed when being diagnosed with a chronic illness such as an **autoimmune disease**. Earlier, the loss of physical health and of the perception of a healthy self was discussed. Loss of the relationship to one's body involves the loss of physical health and of the perception of a healthy self; however, it also includes components of how one experiences their body. Gloria always experienced her body as part of her total being. In her words, there was no separation between her body and her mind; she was just Gloria. After being diagnosed with her **autoimmune disease**, her body became an unwanted, burdensome "other" that no longer felt congruent with her sense of self. Gloria often described herself as "a floating head" as she experienced her "self" as separate from her body. After being diagnosed with her illness, she had to grieve the loss of the positive and loving relationship that she used to have with her body.

This loss and grief are also repeated throughout the course of the patient's illness. As the patient's **autoimmune disease** progresses and evolves, the patient's relationship with their body will likely change multiple times, and some of these moments of change will also be accompanied by grief. Some of these moments of change occur when a patient experiences a lack of control over their body following flare ups. They can also be experienced when medication alters aspects of a patient's body, such as when there is hair loss, weight gain, facial changes, uncontrollable palpitations, and insomnia. All of these are examples of when a patient may experience an overall feeling of loss of control and a painful grief around that aspect of their relationship with their body—a relationship in which they used to feel that they had more of a say.

WORD TO THE WISE

With time, meaning making and reflection, the person can develop new positive relationships to their body. However, it is important that mental health providers do not rush clients through their grief by trying to provide "positive outlooks" and "alternative ways" to experience their bodies before the patient is ready to hear this. Clients need to process their multiple losses in their own way and on their own time and moving too quickly to help them make new relationships with their body can be experienced by the client as another moment of the invisibility of their condition and of its massive impact on their life.

Again, it is important to note that this will not be a one-time grieving process and that offering alternative perspectives will have to occur repeatedly and at various points throughout your work with your client. In the same way that we discuss "loss, grief, and repeat" as a cycle, helping the client make new relationships with their body will also occur in a cycle—loss, make space for grief, present a new perspective, and repeat. How do you know when the client is ready to hear the new perspective? We will get to that a little later on in the section on the stages of mourning.

AND REPEAT AGAIN

As one can imagine, living with an **autoimmune disease** not only costs a person an enormous amount of money but time is also lost. There is the lost time that comes from the potential impact on life expectancy, but there is also time lost due to the many medical and health-related appointments that the person living with the disease attends. This takes away from the patient's professional aspirations and goals, the person's hobbies, and interpersonal relationships. Unfortunately, some relationships will not last through a person's autoimmune diagnosis. Some romantic partners may not understand why their loved one doesn't feel like having sex or doesn't want to make plans too far in advance. Some partners may feel frustrated by the chronicity of the disease and may feel like their loved one is not doing enough to "get better." Some people may feel like they did not sign up to be a caretaker when they entered the romantic relationship and therefore choose to exit the relationship.

The loss of a loved one while trying to manage living with an **autoimmune disease** can be unbearable in some cases and a relief in others, but in either case it can be a great loss. On the one hand, knowing that you lost someone in part because of your illness can be enraging, painful, and can leave you feeling alone to manage your own care, which is hard enough to manage with help. Yet on the other hand, sometimes a person can feel burdened or continuously hurt by a partner who is invalidating and cruel and therefore may feel relief in their absence. In both scenarios, illness is a main contributor to the loss and the patient is left with another experience of mourning.

Sara is a high energy woman in her early thirties. She loves fashion and is always exquisitely dressed from head to toe in the latest trends. When looking at Sara, it is hard to imagine that there are moments when she cannot walk or even get out of bed. Sara was diagnosed with multiple sclerosis when she was 26 and although she receives excellent medical care, she has periods of debilitating flares. Sara was married to her long-term boyfriend shortly after she was diagnosed, and they remained married for four years before divorcing. Sara struggled to stay engaged in conversation and in physically intimate ways with her husband when she was experiencing a flare. She had difficulty concentrating and staying focused, she lacked energy, and she felt depressed. Early on in their relationship her husband tried to be empathic, offering to help Sara with her mobility and being patient when she didn't have energy to interact with him.

However, as the years passed, he began to lose his patience and experienced frustration with her long periods of disengagement. Sara fluctuated between feelings of self-hate, anger at her husband for his lack of empathy, and hope that their relationship could improve. They would frequently argue about how much he was or was not helping Sara when she was not well, whether Sara was "trying enough" to help herself, and whether it made sense for them to stay together. Although they gave couples therapy a try, they ultimately agreed to divorce.

After Sara's divorce she was left feeling enormous grief. She couldn't help but believe that her illness was why her marriage ended. She could entertain the idea that there could have been foundational issues in her marriage to begin with but that did not bring comfort to her. For Sara, her MS was the nail in her marital coffin, and she added this relationship to the list of the losses that MS had brought into her life. Although she was angry with her ex-husband and felt abandoned by him in many ways, she felt like she knew how hard it was for him to live with her. Sara understood how disengaged and low energy she could be when she wasn't feeling well and she was angry that she had no control to change what her body was doing to her in these moments, and that the price was her marriage.

STAGES OF GRIEF: FEELING THE GRIEF MY WAY

The five stages of grief, (denial, anger, bargaining, depression, and acceptance) are well known by most mental health professionals. We also know that these stages do not necessarily occur in this order and that everyone grieves in their own way and time. People who live with **autoimmune diseases** also experience the five stages of grief after being diagnosed with their **autoimmune disease** and throughout living with their illness at various junctures of loss. Again, not everyone will experience all of the five stages of grief or experience them in a particular order. In addition to the five stages, people with **autoimmune disease** typically also experience a strong feeling of guilt as well.

Sara felt great guilt after the loss of her marriage. Initially she experienced a lot of anger towards her husband because she felt like he gave up on her; however, after expressing her anger she was left with a very painful feeling of guilt. Sara blamed herself for the ending of the marriage. She felt that it was illness and her body that created the problems in their relationship, and she fantasized that their relationship would have lasted had it not been for having an **autoimmune disease**. It took Sara months to work through this part of her grief.

Just like when a patient denies the reality of a loss or attempts to bargain with a higher power to undo the loss, a patient will feel guilty about a loss regardless of what others may tell them about how rational or necessary the feeling is. The person will move on from that stage of mourning when they are ready to, and they will transform their feeling of guilt, or denial, or anger, or depression, or bargaining to a more adaptive feeling made of meaning, at their own pace. More will be said on this meaning making process in Chapter 7.

For Sara, a reminder that it was not her fault that her marriage ended did nothing more than make Sara list all the reasons why she believed that it was her fault. Only after Sara was given the space to sit with the pain of her grief in the form of guilt, and have that pain witnessed with nothing more than curiosity, was Sara able to see that the reality was that her marriage had many serious problems that predated her MS diagnosis. She was also able to recognize that her excessive feelings of guilt were also masking a very big pain around how much her MS had cost her and may continue to cost her. This was the moment when she could start beginning to tolerate the pain in a way that could allow for meaning making.

WORD TO THE WISE

One of the most common things I hear from patients regarding their grief is how alone they feel when people rush in to "help them feel better." People who live with **autoimmune disease** are contending with a painful feeling of helplessness to undo the many losses that come from living with their disease. One of the biggest tasks of their mourning process is surrendering to and surviving that immense feeling of helplessness. It is our job as mental health professionals to help them through that by patiently bearing witness to their pain, listening with curiosity, and trusting yourself as the provider to know when it is the right time to begin introducing possibilities for hope. You will notice a shift in how the patient talks about their losses. At first, patients will likely want to tell you about their losses and want you to be listening and helping them contain their grief. Each patient will do this on their own time, but at some point, you will likely hear some version of "I am so sick of talking about this." This is a cue from the patient that they are likely ready to start making meaning of the loss and to begin finding hope for moving forward despite the loss, and you can be there to help them through that.

4

THE WHEN AND WHAT TO SAY

IT IS A Monday morning on a crowded subway cart in New York City. Rosanna, a woman in her twenties living with lupus, is feeling particularly fatigued and achy on this day. At each stop, she meticulously eyes the cart for any potential seats becoming available, but she cannot grab a seat for herself; others are faster. She watches as people give up their seats for pregnant people, senior citizens, and people who are *visibly* differently abled. Rosanna feels very unwell, but she does not feel confident in her ability to advocate for herself at this moment. On the one hand, she thinks about asking someone for their seat and recognizes that it is okay for her to do so; she even thinks about how she could say, "Excuse me, but I am not feeling well. Would you mind if I sat down, please?" On the other hand, she experiences a feeling of shame just when thinking about making this request. She imagines that people might not believe her or that they may look at her in condescending or judgmental ways. Rosanna does not know what would feel worse to her: her physical discomfort or the potentially disapproving gaze of others. Before Rosanna can decide what she wants to do, she has arrived at her stop.

Meanwhile, Vicki was diagnosed with MS when she was 27 years old. To most people she appears to be an able-bodied person but Vicki struggles with walking at times, and in particular she has difficulty going up stairs. One weekend evening, Vicki was at a restaurant and needed to use the restroom. The main restrooms were on the second level of the restaurant and there was one single person restroom on the first floor right next to the hostess' station, that was labeled with a disability sign. Vicki walked slowly up to that restroom and as she reached for the door handle, the hostess said to her, "You can't use that restroom. That is only for people with disabilities. You need to use the restrooms upstairs." Vicki stood and stared at the hostess for a few seconds not knowing what to do. She did not feel like sharing with the hostess that she indeed had a disability and could not walk up the stairs, but she knew that she had to. She looked right at the hostess and said, "You shouldn't make assumptions about people. I have a condition and cannot walk up those stairs." She then opened the bathroom door and walked right in, feeling proud of herself. Vicki shared with me that her thoughts in that moment were that people need to learn that illness and ability do not always look like what people assume them to look like.

This uncertainty around whom to and when to disclose about one's **autoimmune disease** is an extremely common experience for those living with these diseases. Both Rosanna's and Vicki's stories are examples of moments when someone might want to share with a stranger in an effort to advocate for themselves…and/or out of releasing pure frustration. However, as will be discussed, disclosing to loved ones, employers, potential romantic partners, or anyone else one has hopes to have an ongoing relationship with can be even more complicated. In addition to deciding to whom and when to disclose, living with an **autoimmune disease** comes with additional considerations around communicating about one's disease, such as managing people's reactions to you and the illness after having disclosed, navigating communication with one's medical providers, and reflecting on how to communicate to one's children about the illness.

There are so many thoughts that a person who lives with an **autoimmune disease** may juggle when deciding whether to share with someone that they have a chronic illness. For example, first and foremost the person is likely wondering if they will be taken seriously, they may also be wondering if they will be judged or treated negatively in some way, they may worry about losing their autonomy or being pitied, they may be thinking about all the questions that they might hear from the other person, and they may worry that the other person may no longer see them as competent. Sharing with family members can be difficult enough and those will carry different considerations from disclosing to an employer, child, or potential romantic partner...so let's talk about them!

TOO MUCH OR NOT ENOUGH: FAMILY

Many years ago, while I was still a graduate student, I briefly spoke to a young woman with Crohn's disease. This person's illness had progressed into a severe case, and she had been hospitalized multiple times. It was during one of these hospitalizations that she told me that she struggled to work on some days because she felt so ill, and that her mother told her that there wasn't anything actually wrong with her and that she just needed to "suck it up and get over it." This is clearly an example of insufficient empathy on this mother's part, and a moment of invisibility of this young woman's illness. Unfortunately, as I have been describing throughout this book, this is not uncommon when it comes to **autoimmune diseases**, even when the diseases are so severe that they warrant hospitalization. In some cases, family members do not want their loved ones to be sick, which sometimes can be the driver of their denial and lack of empathy.

However, at times family may also not want to acknowledge the reality of the fragility of the human body and of life, and how much of it we as humans cannot control. For some family members it can be easier to deny their loved ones' condition than to face the reality that sometimes people get sick and die, and there is nothing we can do to stop it. If this unempathetic reaction is what a person living with an **autoimmune disease** receives from a loved one, they may regret having disclosed their illness. Unfortunately, in many cases one cannot predict how their family will react, and one cannot always hide the impact of their illness on their daily life from the people that they live with.

On the flip side, some family members may be excessively concerned with their loved ones' health, offering help in a manner that leaves the person living with the illness feeling overly dependent on others and invisible in a different way. Susie, a patient with severe lupus, talks about how she is often frustrated by her mother's rush to help her walk or to tackle a task. Although Susie often appreciates her mother's help, she doesn't like to feel like she cannot do things on her own and in moments feels unheard when her mother insists on helping even though Susie does not want any assistance. Additionally, this kind of excessive concern may make it less likely that the person living with the illness will ask for help. Even in moments when Susie needed help and wanted it, she stopped asking for it from her mother because she didn't want to encourage her mother's intrusive insistence on helping. For Susie and for others, this dynamic can become a situation where the patient regrets disclosing their illness to their family. There is so much already out of one's control when living with an **autoimmune disease**, so family being overly involved in a person's care can make it feel like the person with the illness has even less control than they actually have, and as you can imagine this does not feel good!

Again, it is hard to predict how others will react. The hope for many people living with **autoimmune disease** is that family members will be supportive and provide care, but that they will also listen to and hear the person's needs and not criticize or infantilize. This would be the benefit of sharing about one's **autoimmune disease** with one's family members. Family members can also become **autoimmune disease** activists and can help spread awareness and education about these diseases, which can be experienced by many **autoimmune disease** patients as empowering. Family can help practically as well, taking on things like preparing meals and running errands when their loved one doesn't feel up to the task, providing financial assistance when needed, accompanying their loved one to medical appointments, and being a supportive ear when needed. For some patients with **autoimmune disease**, there can be many benefits to sharing with family about one's illness.

WILL I BE TREATED DIFFERENTLY OR LEFT OUT COMPLETELY?

Many people who live with **autoimmune diseases** require accommodations in order to carry out their responsibilities in the workplace, whether it be flexible hours to help manage varying energy levels throughout the day, or access to joint-friendly workplace equipment for those with arthritis and joint pain. However, many people with **autoimmune disease** do not feel comfortable sharing with their employer that they have a disability and require accommodation. Many people who live with **autoimmune disease** fear that disclosing their illness will result in exclusion and discrimination, and at times their fear may be warranted.

Most of us are familiar with the power of implicit bias. Well-meaning employers will encourage their employees to speak openly about their disabilities and needs, and these employers may very well believe that they want to help their employees with their disabilities in the workplace. Yet not all employers are aware of or educated on implicit bias or what their implicit biases are regarding people with disabilities. Knowing that an employee has a disability will likely tap into these biases and if the employer is not aware of them, they may end up discriminating inadvertently. There are also the employers who have external bias and are not well-meaning but who on paper have to adhere to the federal and state laws meant to protect those with disability. Such employers can find ways to discriminate if they choose to.

For example, according to the American Disabilities Act (ADA) of 1990, employers are required to provide "reasonable accommodations" to "qualified employees" with disabilities to assist them with meeting the requirements of their job. However, the employer is not required to provide accommodations to the person with the disability if the accommodation creates "undue hardship" for the company. Even though they would have to prove it, the employer could easily make this claim if they wanted to. It is important to note that realistically there are ways to get around laws that are meant to protect people, resulting in discrimination and inequity. Additionally, a person with an **autoimmune disease** who chooses to disclose their illness to an employer may be protected by law one day but may find themselves without that protection if a law is unexpectedly amended in the future.

Many people who live with **autoimmune disease**, for all of the reasons just mentioned, choose not to disclose their illness to their employer. As you can imagine, they fear being passed over for opportunities, not being taken as seriously as their peers, losing their job and the income and health insurance that comes with it, or generally being treated differently. On the flip side, not disclosing means absence of accommodations and this can negatively impact the person's quality of life, productivity, and in effect, professional advancement. For example, a Lupus Foundation of America survey found 55 percent of lupus patients reported a complete or partial loss of their income because they no longer are able to work full time. One in three have been temporarily disabled by the disease, and one in four currently receive disability payments (Lupus Foundation of America, 2024). Other research found that the combination of the invisibility of the disease, the fluctuating condition, and a lack of understanding by employers explains why many patients with **autoimmune disease** are unable to work, and they conclude that more data is needed to inform workplace adjustments for this population (Booth, et al., 2018).

Clearly if this group of the working force is going to be able to do their jobs there is a great need for increased accommodation. Yet the reality is that people are sometimes understandably too afraid to disclose and a part of that is that employers do not always foster an environment where one would feel safe disclosing, or they may directly or implicitly communicate that requesting accommodations is not something to be encouraged. In some of these cases, people who do not feel comfortable disclosing in one work setting may feel more comfortable seeking new employment in an environment where they do feel safe in sharing about their illness and feel supported with respect to their needs.

AM I WORTH IT?

One of the most common assumptions that people who live with **autoimmune diseases** make is that nobody would want to have a romantic relationship with them if they knew about their illness. This is a reasonable concern as the reality is that there are some people who would not want to be romantically involved with someone who has a debilitating chronic illness. However, that does not mean that a romantic relationship is not possible when living with an **autoimmune disease**.

Donna started dating Andre for a little over three months before she was diagnosed with lupus. The relationship had been going very well, and she felt like if things continued at this pace, they could find themselves in a very serious relationship. During this three-month period, as Donna and Andre were getting to know each other, she began to have significant joint pain, joint swelling, and fatigue, which led her to see a PCP who referred her to a rheumatologist. Donna was quickly diagnosed with lupus. As she went through this process of receiving her diagnosis, she started to have fears that Andre would leave her and would experience her as a burden. She was astonished when Andre expressed a desire to help her share the news of the diagnosis with her family and continued to date her as if nothing had changed. Fifteen years later, Donna and Andre are still together, married, and have two dogs. Andre is still as loving and supportive of Donna as he was when they first learned about her illness.

Not all relationships end like Donna's. Some partners do feel overwhelmed by the situation and ultimately end the relationship. Some partners stay in the relationship, but cannot tolerate the hardships that come with having a partner who lives with a chronic illness. In such cases, there is often a lot of conflict that can lead to an ending of the relationship. Some patients who live with **autoimmune disease** repeatedly question, "Am I worth it?" when they think about what comes with having a romantic relationship with them.

In Donna's situation, Andre already knew about her diagnosis since they had started dating prior to her receiving the diagnosis, and therefore Donna was not tasked with the decision of whether to disclose or not. Many people who live with **autoimmune diseases**, however, do need to make this decision when they want to date or pursue romantic relationships. Some people share that they have a chronic illness very early on in a relationship, before there is a strong attachment. This is done to protect themselves in case the relationship ends following the disclosure. Other people wait until they really trust someone before telling them about their **autoimmune disease**, and some people hide it from their partners for years, until it can no longer be hidden.

WHAT DO I TELL MY CHILDREN?

The decision of how and when to share one's diagnosis with one's children is one that is extremely difficult for people who live with **autoimmune**

disease. Parents who live with **autoimmune diseases** often feel forced to think about how much to explain to their children about what their disease is. Many parents worry about scaring their children and creating worries for them around illness and mortality. On the other hand, living with an **autoimmune disease** is something that is very difficult to hide from others when living in the same home, and especially from children who often demand a lot of energy from their parents.

Some parents whose illnesses predate the birth of their children feel that it is easier to talk about the disease in a way that normalizes it, starting at a very young age given that it is something that will be a part of their children's lives from birth. For example, a mother who has lupus may say to their three-year-old child who wants to run outside in the sun, "Mommy can't run in the sun because of lupus but mommy can run in the shade under the trees with you." Additionally, parents who have **autoimmune diseases** typically need a lot of rest. This is also something that some parents may wish to explain to their children early on. Other parents may prefer to avoid having these discussions with their children for as long as possible. They at times worry about disrupting their children's lives. They may also fear the stress that could come with having to manage the reactions that their children may have to learning about their parent's diagnosis. For example, after sharing with their children, some children may fear that they will get sick too, a fear that many parents who have **autoimmune disease** have themselves.

Something for mental health professionals to be aware of is that one of the most frightening thoughts for parents who have an **autoimmune disease** is that their child will inherit it. Parents may also fear that if their children know about their illness, they may not perceive them in a favorable way or as their "hero." As is easy to imagine, this could feel like a very painful loss for a parent.

WHAT SHOULD I DO?

One of the best ways of helping clients cope with potential reactions from others is by being educated on the most common types of unhelpful reactions that they will likely receive after disclosing. Preparing our clients for what they may expect from others and then making space to explore how to handle each of the possible reactions may help our clients feel more confident in their decision of whether to disclose or not. The range of reactions that people may have when learning about someone's **autoimmune disease** is infinite; however, there are four unhelpful reactions that people with **autoimmune disease** frequently report encountering after having disclosed. Let us explore them.

Jenny had been feeling ill for a very long time and although she was deeply frightened when she learned that she had Hashimoto's disease, she also felt a sense of relief that she now had a label to describe her experience. Even though she would have to take medication for the rest of her life, she was glad that it would help her to feel better. Jenny was eager to share this life changing news with her best friend, Candice.

After meeting Candice at a coffee shop, Jenny told Candice that she had some important news that she wanted to share with her. She told Candice that she was diagnosed with Hashimoto's disease. Almost immediately after she shared this, Candice began to sob uncontrollably. Candice said, "How can this happen? How can this be? What are we going to do? This is terrible." Jenny felt awful, as if she had done something to hurt Candice. Jenny found herself hugging Candice and comforting her, telling her that she would be fine and not to worry about her. Jenny thought about the ways that Candice tends to make things about herself, even when they are not about her. She wished that she had thought about that before sharing this news with her.

Candice's reaction is an example of the first of the four common unhelpful reactions people will likely experience after disclosing that they have an **autoimmune disease**. This is what I call the "Needy Other Reaction." This is a situation in which the person receiving the information about the illness reacts in a way that communicates that they need comforting. In these moments, the needs of the person who has the **autoimmune disease** take a back seat, leaving their experience invisible. Witnessing this reaction and the subsequent management of the other person's emotional needs can feel exhausting for the person who is living with the illness and oftentimes will discourage them from wanting to disclose again. Although this reaction can feel like a disappointing shock initially, most of the time it is consistent with how the person who is reacting tends to react in other situations, as Jenny noted about Candice.

WORD TO THE WISE

This is something mental health professionals can encourage their clients to keep in mind when considering disclosure. They can think about who they want to share with and what that person is typically like when they receive emotionally laden information. This is a useful thing to think about in general when exploring with your clients whether they want to disclose or not.

The second common unhelpful reaction is the "No Big Deal" reaction, which can often be experienced by a person with an **autoimmune disease** as extremely hurtful and at times even violent. Chris had type I diabetes and wanted to share it with their father, hoping to receive some support. Chris' father heard Chris share and then immediately replied with, "What are you worried about? That is no big deal. You'll take some meds and be fine." Others may react with, "Why are you crying? You are really overreacting. Get over it already." This type of reaction is a great mismatch from what the person living with the

autoimmune disease is probably feeling. In all likelihood, the person living with the disease would not be sharing this information if it wasn't a "big deal," and may also be feeling frightened and uncertain about their future. This "No Big Deal" reaction can leave the person who shared feeling deeply alone and confused about their own experience of what is happening to them emotionally and physically. They may even feel punished for sharing, forced to hold their experience alone, and invisible once again.

The "Psychologically Abusive Reaction" is another reaction that people who have **autoimmune disease** may experience when sharing. Although this is a reaction that people who live with other forms of illness, such as heart disease or cancer may hear, I believe that people who live with **autoimmune disease** may hear it a little more often because of society's general unfamiliarity with these diseases. There is a general lack of awareness around the seriousness of **autoimmune disease** and the impact on quality of life, as well as public unfamiliarity with the etiology and prognosis of these diseases. This general ignorance can be heard in this type of reaction in blaming phrases like, "You did this to yourself. You feel sick because you spent too much time in the sun as a teenager. You should've listened to me when I told you that was bad for you." This type of reaction can also take the form of blatant verbal abuse such as, "Of course your joints hurt, you are fat. Maybe try losing some weight and you'll feel better" or "You aren't sick, you are just lazy. You think you are going to find an excuse not to do things? I am not going to be fooled by you." Most frequently, this reaction comes in the form of the phrase, "But you don't look sick," which is a passive aggressive version of this reaction as it implies that the person with the illness is being dishonest in some way or is not to be believed.

These types of experiences are certainly the "kicking me when I am already down" kind and as can be imagined, can be extremely harmful to the person who is living with the **autoimmune disease**. Not only may this type of reaction impact the person's sense of self-worth, but it may also impact their willingness to seek treatment, adhere to medication regimens, and may result in the person with the illness pushing themselves beyond what is healthy for their body at a given time.

WORD TO THE WISE

As awful as these abusive reactions are, in my experience I have found that they are surprisingly more common than one may think. As previously noted, although typically people tend to react as you would expect them to, oftentimes this abusive reaction comes to many as a surprise. People who one may not expect to react in an abusive way may do so, especially when it comes to the "but you don't look sick" comment. Most of the time, these abusive and toxic reactions are emotionally unregulated attempts to find an explanation for and a solution to a loved one's illness. This doesn't excuse the abusive behavior, but I share this to drive home why these reactions may be so common when a person who has an **autoimmune disease** shares. There are of course situations in which someone is just being straight up abusive because they are an abusive person and there is no underlying concern for the person sharing about their illness. As I imagine you would suspect, in these situations it is better for the person with the illness to not share anything vulnerable with the abusive person.

The last of the most common unhelpful reactions is the "Patronizing Narrative." This reaction is one in which the person's subjective experience is hijacked after sharing. This occurs when the person living with **autoimmune disease** is spoken to in a patronizing manner that ignores their actual experience and elevates hearsay or other people's experiences of the illness. For example, after sharing about their illness, a person may hope to hear the following questions: "How are you feeling about this diagnosis?" or "what do the doctors say about your prognosis or how it will impact on your life?" However, what they hear instead is something like, "Oh, my friend's cousin had something like that, and it was so hard because she couldn't work anymore. You poor thing, it is going to be so terrible." This reaction can also take the form of, "It's going to be okay. My uncle's coworker has an **autoimmune disease**, and she is totally fine." The two forms of the reaction are different from each other but they both take on an all-knowing patronizing tone that objectifies the person with the illness and doesn't allow space for their actual unique and subjective experience. Once again this could be a moment where the person living with the disease feels invisible.

Although these common reactions can feel unwanted, unpleasant, awful and hurtful, most of the time this is not the intention of the people who are reacting. Chronic illness can be a very anxiety provoking topic and unless you have experienced chronic illness intimately in your own life (and even not always then), it may be difficult figuring out how to react. The person reacting could be managing multiple feelings, such as their worry about the person with the illness, their own anxieties about their body's fragility and future mortality, and sorting through how to be most helpful, among other worries and emotions.

This is one reason why even though these reactions often make people with **autoimmune disease** want to share less, it is important for our clients to think about how they can talk to the people in their lives about how certain reactions make them feel. In many cases there is space for growth. Having the people in the patient's life have a better understanding of what it means to live with an **autoimmune disease** may allow for them to be of help to the person in a way that the person actually wants and needs. We as clinicians can help our clients recognize that the people in our life may just "not get it" and that with some patience and education, perhaps they may learn to "get it" more and more. This is an excellent exercise that can start with people's initial reactions to receiving the news that their loved one has an **autoimmune disease**.

As discussed earlier in this chapter, moments of potential disclosure will occur again and again throughout the lives of people who live with **autoimmune diseases**, therefore there will be ample opportunities for practicing this exercise. The earlier this practice begins, the better. Again, if there is a situation in which a person is just flat out abusive, then of course this difficult work of educating and sharing about how it feels to live with **autoimmune disease** is too vulnerable. This exercise would not apply, and it is unlikely that the abusive person's attitude would change.

COMMUNICATION WITH HEALTHCARE PROFESSIONALS

One may imagine that communication about **autoimmune disease** with one's healthcare providers would be less complicated for patients than communicating with lay people given that healthcare providers know what these diseases are. This is not necessarily the case. Oftentimes, physicians are using labs and scans to assess improvement or worsening of one's condition and when it comes to **autoimmune disease**, the symptoms that the labs and scans correspond to are not always the symptoms that cause the patient the most distress, and vice versa. For example, according to LupusUK.org, between 80–90 percent of patients who have lupus report that fatigue is their most debilitating symptom. Unfortunately, fatigue levels do not tend to correlate with disease markers of activity (i.e. blood work) and increases in medication seem to have little benefit when it comes to reducing levels of fatigue (LupusUK. org). This can be quite frustrating for patients when according to their doctors they are "doing better" but they may continue to feel unwell and unable to engage in daily activities. In these situations, patients may feel misunderstood or like their doctors do not believe them when they say they are not feeling better. This is another example of invisibility.

Similarly, there is variation between physicians and patients regarding what constitutes health. This can be the case when a patient feels that they are improving but a doctor sees no evidence for this in measures of disease activity. For example, in her co-authored book *If You Have to Wear an Ugly Dress, Learn to Accessorize* (McNamara & Kemper, 2011), Karen Kemper, a scleroderma patient, speaks about the incongruities between how she feels she is doing and her doctor's perspective on how she is feeling. She recounts an incident where her doctor asked her how she is feeling, and she said she was feeling better. Her physician then turned to the medical student in the room and said, "She always thinks she is better." Karen then spoke about how her doctor doesn't experience her as getting better because her disease progression continues; however, Karen's assessment is not based on the medical indicators of her disease progression but more on her current ability to adapt to the disease in a way that allows her to enjoy her life. She stated, "I was looking at it in terms of function and feeling. My doctor was looking at it in terms of presence or absence of disease and symptoms." (McNamara & Kemper, 2011, p. 104).

WORD TO THE WISE

These potential mismatches between what a patient and doctor experience are very important to explore with our clients. Some patients may not feel confident or comfortable letting their doctors know what symptoms concern them the most because they fear being dismissed. In many cases, patients have had the experience of being dismissed in past encounters with their providers. This doesn't mean that what the physicians are measuring isn't also important. What it *does* mean is that there must also be space for patients to be able to let their doctors know what they would really like the most help with. It is our job as mental health professionals to help our clients work up to advocating for themselves during their medical appointments.

Unfortunately, doctors will not always have answers for how to help patients with these symptoms, just like when it comes to fatigue as previously mentioned. However, it is still critical that we work with our clients to encourage them to continue to try to ask for what they need so that they do not default to a position of passivity, hopelessness, and invisibility, or stop asking questions completely. Sometimes doctors may not have the answers and sometimes they will, but if patients stop asking questions, they may miss out on opportunities that may bring them relief. Our clients do not have to feel helpless or invisible when doctors do not have the answers. In those moments, our job as clinicians is to help our clients attempt to feel heard and understood, and to adapt to whatever challenge they are facing in a way that will help them feel joy in their life and a sense of empowerment-- even if the empowerment doesn't come from getting the answers they seek.

Additional communication frustrations for patients with **autoimmune diseases** also emerge when patients are seeing both medical doctors and alternative providers, which is often the case for most patients with **autoimmune disease**. Patients may also be working with homeopathic doctors, licensed acupuncturists, body-work healers, and other alternative providers. As discussed, medical doctors may not always have the answers to what patients are looking for. Patients search for answers to these questions with alternative providers, and many find alternative healing quite helpful when it comes to managing day to day symptoms or coping with the stress that comes with having an **autoimmune disease**.

Problems may emerge however when one's medical doctors and one's alternative healers provide conflicting information. This can be confusing and upsetting for patients. As mental health professionals, we can assist our clients in identifying which perspective has empirical support, what helps them feel better, and how to comfortably assert their needs to both types of providers. Because many alternative healers are not regulated by any licensing board, it is imperative that patients be able to assess whether an alternative healer's suggestion could be harmful. Therefore, patients should be encouraged to ask their medical physicians if what they are doing is safe.

Some medical professionals may not believe alternative therapies are useful, but they may not take issue with patients exploring them. Therefore, it is important for patients to feel like they have chosen medical doctors who will support their need to explore other therapies, so that the patient can feel safe enough to speak freely with their doctor about what these alternative therapies constitute. Our role as mental health professionals is to encourage our clients to think very deeply about their relationship with their medical doctors, and to support them in establishing relationships with physicians who they feel listen to them, take them seriously, and make time for them.

Lastly, it is important to help our patients recognize that their medical doctors are just people like everybody else and that they too may say well-intentioned things at times that could be hurtful. One time I came back from a vacation and my rheumatologist at the time asked, "Why don't you have a tan?" My immediate reaction was one of confusion and frustration as he was the one who told me to stay out of the sun. I pointed that out to him, and he acknowledged that he wasn't thinking at that moment and that I was absolutely right to stay out of the sun. This wasn't the first time or the last time that my doctor said something that was hurtful. This is the case for most patients.

Luckily, I was able to advocate for myself by communicating to my doctor how he was giving me mixed messages about what I should be doing to care for myself. This example of self-advocacy is what we as mental health clinicians need to help our patients with. It may sound very simple, but it is extremely difficult for many people to do. Being a patient as we know is very vulnerable and especially in medical settings where doctors are not always trained in the art of bedside manner, patients are often in gowns or scantily clothed, and the uneven distribution of power is directly evident. We can encourage our patients to bring lists of questions to their doctor, ask that they discuss their treatment goals only after they have changed back into their regular clothes and are out of the gown, and work with our patients on assertiveness skills so that they can start to feel more confident advocating for themselves in medical settings.

WORD TO THE WISE

People are going to say hurtful things. Most of the time not because they want to hurt the person who is living with the **autoimmune disease**. As discussed earlier in this chapter, most of the time it comes from a place of ignorance or emotional dysregulation, sometimes it comes from not understanding what feels like care and what doesn't, and other times it is just a regretful mistake. It can be very easy for patients to walk around angry and feeling misunderstood every day. We mental health professionals can explore with our clients how to extend some grace to the people in their lives just as they would like others to extend to them. We also need to encourage our clients to directly communicate their needs to the people in their lives and to explicitly state what is and what is not helpful. This communication serves as advocacy for the patient and for patients with **autoimmune disease** in general.

For our clients who live with **autoimmune disease**, what is helpful and what is not helpful may be obvious because they are the ones with the lived experience of what it is like to live with this type of illness. This is not true for everyone else. These diseases and how they impact a person's life are completely foreign to most people, likely even to you as a clinician. Until I was diagnosed with lupus, I had never heard of it before, and although I had heard of rheumatoid arthritis in my early adulthood, I had no idea that it was an **autoimmune disease** or knew what **autoimmune diseases** were at all. I assumed it was something elderly people were diagnosed with. I am sure I am not unique in that experience. Extending a little grace, being curious about others' reactions, and direct communication will go a long way for our clients in helping them feel a little less invisible.

5

COMMON DEFENSES & REACTIONS

EVERYONE REACTS TO receiving an **autoimmune disease** diagnosis in their own way but there are some defenses and reactions that are commonly observed in clients with **autoimmune diseases**. These are denial, avoidance, manic defense, shame, dissociation, symbolization through behaviors, depression, and anxiety. Often these defenses and reactions present temporarily as a person attempts to cope with receiving a diagnosis and during periods of subsequent adjustment, such as a bad flare up or change in the status of a significant relationship. A person's health is extremely likely to be negatively impacted when they remain stuck in any one of these defensive or reactionary states. As mental health providers, we can help our clients to identify when they are experiencing these states. We can then work with them to process the feelings underlying these states and help them to mourn what has been lost and to accept the realities of what it means to live with an **autoimmune disease**.

DENIAL AND AVOIDANCE

Xiamara had been an active 25-year-old until she began to have tingling sensations in her legs for a few months, which then worsened leaving her with difficulty walking. She also found herself feeling "foggy-headed" and frequently fatigued. Xiamara was referred to a neurologist by her PCP and was subsequently diagnosed with multiple sclerosis. She began treatment and her neurologist informed her that she would need to slow down her very active lifestyle, at least until she was feeling better for a consistent period. She was also instructed on how to take her medication and on the importance of taking it exactly as directed.

Although multiple sclerosis is a life changing disease, Xiamara did not recognize this upon diagnosis. In fact, for the first six months post diagnosis, she appeared to behave as if nothing had changed in her life at all. She continued to work long hours, go out late at night with friends, and not allow herself enough time for rest. Her parents were concerned about her and reminded her that she could flare if she didn't take good care of herself. Xiamara shirked their concern and would tell them that she was "fine." This denial of the seriousness of her condition also impacted on the consistency with which she took her medication. She frequently avoided taking her medication if she was having a particularly good day with respect to how she felt in her body. Unfortunately, after several months of denying the reality and impact of her illness, and avoiding treatments, Xiamara had a very bad flare. She presented for psychotherapy following this flare. She shared that she wanted help with facing the reality of her illness because she was struggling to do that on her own, and even though she knew her family wanted to help, their comments often made her angry.

As mental health professionals we know that it is important to think about what it is that our clients are denying and why. On the surface we can say that a client is avoiding their medication and their self-care because they are denying that there is an actual medical concern. However, as we can all imagine and as we see in the interaction between Xiamara and her family, simply pointing that out to the client is not going to be very effective in changing the client's behaviors. In fact, similar to Xiamara's reaction, people who live with **autoimmune disease** are likely to feel frustrated, angry, and misunderstood when loved ones suggest that they take better care of themselves. We as providers will not make this same mistake! If we think about what lies underneath the client's denial and avoidance, we can better understand that what the client is avoiding is confronting their feelings of sadness around the multiple losses that come with the reality of being diagnosed with an **autoimmune disease**. The client is denying the need to have to mourn. So you will have to work with the client slowly and gently to help them identify these avoided feelings.

MANIC DEFENSE

The manic defense is a particular version or manifestation of denial where a person engages in overactivity in an effort to not have to deal with feelings associated with the reality of a situation. People who live with **autoimmune disease** may exhibit this defense when wanting to prove to oneself that nothing has changed about their life. For example, a patient who may need to get a lot of rest to avoid a flare may make social plans every night of the week without a break between work and social outing, insisting that they are fine but then crashing on the weekend, only to repeat this cycle again the following week until eventually landing in the hospital. Another patient may become obsessed with training for a marathon in order to prove that nothing has changed. When a client is engaging in manic defense, time and space are overly filled and there is no space and time to identify, feel, or process emotions. Like denial, this is another form of avoidance.

WORD TO THE WISE

Similar to denial, trying to confront the client with what they are doing in using this defense will likely just upset them. You may come off as unsupportive as the client is not ready to create a space and sit in it with you to explore their reaction. You must wait for the space and time to present itself, and it will when the client crashes from exhaustion. This will be a natural opening of space. At this moment, you will have an opportunity to non-judgmentally ask the client to be curious about what they imagine may have contributed to the crash. Build on their answers and they will eventually see that they have been physically overdoing it. Then there can be space to think about the, "Why that might be?" and the avoided feelings will slowly begin to emerge.

SHAME

One of the most common reactions to receiving an autoimmune diagnosis is shame. There are various reasons for this reaction. For example, people who may be used to being extremely reliable or high achieving may not be able to meet a professional deadline or may have to cancel plans. They may feel ashamed of the physical limitations that their illness puts on them and the way in which it impacts on their responsibilities. People may also be ashamed to even share the reason why they had to miss their deadline or cancel. They may experience sharing their diagnosis with others and identifying it as the reason for not being able to follow through with a responsibility as an "excuse."

Others may feel ashamed of the particular symptoms of their illness. For example, some **autoimmune diseases** create gynecological symptoms such as vaginal sores, which some patients may feel ashamed of, and which may impact on their sexual relationships. There are also some **autoimmune diseases** that can create scarring on the face, can cause skin discoloration, significant hair loss, and rashes. Whether or not it is accurate, some patients with **autoimmune disease** may also feel shame if they feel that they played some role in the development of their disease. A patient may also feel ashamed that they did not engage in physical exercises regularly, had a poor diet, or partook in frequent drug use.

It can be quite challenging for a clinician to help a client with **autoimmune disease** work through their shame because shame influences a person's willingness to share vulnerably and honestly with others. Therefore, it can take quite a bit of time for a client with an **autoimmune disease** to open up about their feelings of shame and what they may feel ashamed of. A very good place to start is for the client to be able to identify that shame is indeed something that they experience in relation to their **autoimmune disease**.

Once that is acknowledged, space has opened up to explore the shame. Stay away from directly asking a client if they feel shame, and rather track for moments of shame in the client's body language or verbal expression that you can then very gently comment on. For example, a client may be speaking about how they can no longer help their elderly family member with grocery shopping, and you notice that they glance down and physically shrink into the couch. You may want to comment with, "You look like you have a strong feeling about that," and then see how the client responds. Over time, as the client feels more trusting of you, they will likely talk more about their shame, and you will have an opportunity to help them make peace with not being able to control the uncontrollable that is embedded within their shame.

DISSOCIATION AND SYMBOLIZATION THROUGH BEHAVIORS

Recent studies (e.g. Macarenco, Opariuc-Dan, & Nedelcea, 2021; Gupta et al., 2017; Yildirim, et al., 2020) have been examining the role of dissociation and alexithymia in **autoimmune diseases**. This area of research has developed as an extension of the relationship between trauma and **autoimmune disease**. The results of this body of research are mixed and it is difficult to identify the specific pathways and effects of trauma, dissociation, and alexithymia on **autoimmune disease**, and/

or how each of these factors impact the others or if and how they each mediate or moderate the **autoimmune disease**. What we do know is that dissociation and alexithymia (difficulty identifying and verbalizing feelings) often present in clients with **autoimmune disease**.

As clinicians, we know that dissociation is a defense mechanism in which conscious awareness of an experience is altered. This alteration can be experienced in a variety of ways ranging from mild, such as day-dreaming, briefly "spacing out," or forgetting something just heard, to more serious such as depersonalization, derealization, or amnesia. We also know that both content and affect associated with an experience can be dissociated. When content is dissociated important facts are omitted from a narrative, appearing to have been, but are not necessarily, forgotten.

For example, a client may tell you their entire medical history and leave out telling you about a major surgery that they had but then are able to recall the surgery when their partner reminds them of it. When working with clients who have **autoimmune disease**, it is important for clinicians to be cognizant of the possible presence of dissociation of affect, which occurs when a person's affect does not match the content of what is being shared. An example of this is when a client may be speaking about a very frightening situation, but their emotional expression is not one that would signal an experience of fear. There is a disconnect between what you see in the client's face and body language from the content of what they are sharing.

It is especially important for clinicians to be on the lookout for this when a client is discussing difficult experiences related to living with their **autoimmune disease**. The use of dissociation as a defense mechanism is different from the use of denial in that there is no active attempt to avoid verbally addressing something difficult to accept. In fact, when it comes to experiencing dissociated affect, the client may actually be able to talk about objectively difficult components that accompany living with an **autoimmune disease**, unlike with denial where the client may very quickly want to shut the conversation down (e.g. "I am fine. It's not a big deal. I don't need medication"). When it comes to dissociation, clients living with **autoimmune disease** will likely talk to you about very painful procedures, traumatic medical interventions, losses, and daily difficulties but without commensurate affect. Their affect may be neutral or very muted and it is unlikely that unprompted they will tell you what they feel.

WORD TO THE WISE

A complicating factor is the similarity between presentations of dissociation as a defense mechanism with the cognitive dysfunction of "brain fog," as it is colloquially referred to. Brain fog is a symptom that can occur in people who have **autoimmune disease** due to inflammation of the nervous system, including the brain and the spinal cord, and due to abnormalities in blood flow to certain parts of the brain. Brain fog can include forgetfulness, problems with word finding, and difficulty concentrating and attending, which can present like dissociation. It is critical that we take our clients seriously when they say that they are experiencing brain fog and that we do not quickly assume that they are defensively dissociating.

One may wonder how we can go about telling the difference. The truth is that we may not always be able to; however, there are some things to consider. Brain fog will typically accompany a flare up, so it will likely present with other **autoimmune disease** symptoms. Again, this may not always occur but commonly does. Another thing is that severe inflammation of the nervous system can be seen on an MRI. Unfortunately, milder versions may not always be visible. Additionally, abnormalities of blood flow can be identified using SPECT scans. A more easily observable way to distinguish between defensive dissociation and brain fog is that when a person frequently uses dissociation as a defense mechanism, communication and symbolization will tend to occur through behaviors rather than with words.

Regardless of whether a client is experiencing brain fog or dissociation, they will likely be having difficulty identifying and naming their feelings. We as mental health clinicians can work with our clients to connect to what they are feeling and to verbalize what is either defensively dissociated or difficult to access due to brain fog. The hope is that if our clients experience a greater understanding of what they are feeling and can then begin to process those feelings, they will then be more likely to adhere to their medication and to engage in behavioral changes that could be helpful to them overall.

Interestingly, there is some research (Lumley et al., 2007) that has found a correlation (likely mediated by childhood trauma) between alexithymia and altered autonomic, endocrine, and immune activity leading to tissue damage and therefore negatively contributing to any potential inflammatory process. As discussed in Chapter 2, we know that trauma is not the sole contributor to **autoimmune diseases** and psychotherapy is not its cure; however, we do know that psychotherapy helps improve clients' reported quality of life as it relates to the disease. Although verbalizing feelings is not the cure for these diseases, perhaps identification and verbalization of feelings and connection to commensurate affect may moderate one of the many factors that contribute to organ inflammation. I am not aware of any evidence for this at this time but as I imagine you do; I have experience with clients who self-report "feeling better" after being able to identify and verbalize their feelings. Usually, the client means that they are feeling emotionally better, but I have noticed other changes in these moments. Clients look like they have more energy and speak and move with more fluidity.

Janina has been living with undiagnosed autoimmune symptoms since her adolescence. She had visited the emergency room multiple times in her adolescence for pain in her hips and lower back but was quickly dismissed and told to take pain relievers. Eventually Janina was diagnosed with ankylosing spondylitis, an **autoimmune disease** where tissue hardens mostly in the back and neck but can also affect hips and extremities. Janina was already primed to ignore her feelings as she grew up in a home where she was repeatedly told not to think about what she felt because, "The only thing worth feeling was feeling happy all the time because she was so lucky." Obviously, Janina's privilege did not shield her from the emotional pain of being a human being, yet she buried her feelings to avoid being judged by her family. Her experiences of being dismissed by the medical field did not help with Janina's dissociation.

When I first met Janina, I remember feeling like I was holding a shovel and I needed to dig through massive piles of debris to get to anything that felt like a feeling. Janina struggled to speak in sessions for a long while. She would sit quietly on the couch, looking down and hunching over her legs. I would ask her to tell me how she is feeling, and she would tell me about her physical pain in a very detached manner, as if she was telling me about her grocery list. When I would ask her how she felt about what she was telling me, she would either make gestures or movements with her hands, or she would make unintelligible sounds. Accessing her feelings was very difficult because her feelings were not yet fully formed. She really didn't know what she felt, and her physical gestures and sounds were her attempt to try to start formulating her feelings. They were a form of symbolization.

I would ask Janina what a particular gesture or sound meant, and each time Janina would get a few more words out to describe her feelings. I would also offer some word choices with curiosity when Janina was stuck, and she would tell me if any of those words were reflective of what she was trying to express. Something that was particularly helpful to me was using what I already knew about experiences and feelings that people who live with **autoimmune diseases** commonly have. Having this information helped Janina with feeling understood and seen when she so often felt her experience of her illness was invisible in her family and in past encounters with medical professionals.

DEPRESSION & ANXIETY

I do not think anyone would be surprised to learn that incidence and prevalence of depression and anxiety are extremely high in the population of folks who live with **autoimmune disease**. A mixed-methods large scale international study published in the journal, *Rheumatology*, found that rates of depression and anxiety were significantly higher in the **autoimmune disease** population than in the general population (Sloane et al., 2023). According to the study, 55 percent of **autoimmune disease** participants met criteria for depression compared to 30 percent of the control group, and 57 percent of participants with **autoimmune disease** met criteria for anxiety compared to only 33 percent of the controls. The results of the study also suggest that medical professionals often underestimate the prevalence of depression and anxiety in the **autoimmune disease** population, and that symptoms of anxiety and depression may often be attributed to symptoms of the **autoimmune disease**, such as fatigue or memory problems. A more consistent and thorough screening process for anxiety and depression would be extremely beneficial to patients.

Depression in the **autoimmune disease** population is commonly due to the stressors that come with living with a chronic disease, taking multiple medications, and at times with certain diseases such as lupus, avoiding sunlight. Another contributor is low body image that can accompany weight gain due to certain steroid medications, hair loss, skin changes, or arthritic deformities (Thomas Jr., 2023). Additionally, current ongoing research is exploring whether inflammatory molecules, such as the cytokines interferon alpha, Il-6, and antibody anti-ribosomal-P also contribute to depression (Thomas Jr., 2023) in **autoimmune disease**. Depressed patients are significantly more likely to be non-adherent with their medication regimen, which may lead to medical complications for some patients, therefore it is crucial that depression be treated as soon as possible.

Similar to depression, anxiety often presents in people who live with **autoimmune diseases**, often as a result of the stressors that come with living with a chronic illness. The anxiety is likely to worsen when one's autoimmune symptoms are more severe and then likely subside when the autoimmune symptoms improve. Unlike with depression, inflammation is not understood to be a possible contributor to anxiety in the **autoimmune disease** population. However, like with depression, certain medications such as high doses of steroids, can contribute to anxiety.

As clinicians you are all very familiar with how to work with clients who have depression and anxiety already, so I won't say much about that. However, when working with clients who have **autoimmune disease**, it is also very important to be familiar with the client's medication regimen and their side effects, and to consult with the client's medical doctors if you are not aware of what kinds of side effects are expected. Even if you are informed about a client's medication and what a typical reaction is, it is still a good idea to inquire with the client's medical doctor about any other possible explanations for a client's depressed mood or anxiety. For example, could their anxiety be an indication of a rising flare that requires medical attention? Sometimes something can be adjusted medically that can improve a patient's mood and other times there is no alternative.

Nevertheless, as their therapist you can address clients' depression and anxiety, and as will be discussed in Chapter 8, work with clients to adapt to their circumstances and create meaning out of their illness.

6

SO LONG AND HELLO

GREW UP SPENDING the entire summer on the beaches of Greece. I loved the dark bronze tan that I would have by the end of the summer, the freedom of running on the shore all day with the friends that I only got to see during this time of year, the carefreeness of jumping in for a swim, and the utter happiness that I felt in those moments. These experiences are especially important to me as they are associated with relationships that meaningfully shaped the person that I am. After thirty years, they became more than just experiences. They are a part of me, a part of my identity. I could never have imagined it being any other way. I was crushed when during my first rheumatology appointment my doctor said that I would have to stay out of the sun, wear sunblock, long sleeves, and a hat. I immediately started to think about my summers. What would I do? How would I be with my friends? Would I still be able to enjoy the beach? Would people stare at me? Would I have to explain why I looked like a beekeeper?

Perhaps this sounds dramatic or trite. I can imagine some people thinking that I should have just been happy that I wasn't going to die. I certainly was happy about that, but I also felt like I was saying, "So long!" to a very important part of me. A specific part of me was born from those repeated experiences on the beach. It was as if a piece of me was being restricted, and I didn't know what would happen to it. Would it disappear? Would I find another way of expressing that part of myself?

I was really frightened. It truly felt like a loss. I never had those same beach experiences again.

Since the time of my diagnosis in 2010, I have had to create a specific routine for dealing with the sun, which sets in motion as soon as spring starts and in which I engage in until summer ends. The impact of the sun on my health does not only affect me when at the beach. I need to protect myself any time that I am outdoors and in the sun. That means that any time I take a walk or go to an outdoor café or a park, I need to wear all my protective gear (i.e. hat, sunscreen, cover up with long sleeves) if there isn't ample shade. The necessity to protect myself from the sun has certainly changed an aspect of my life. It has been an experience of both loss and of inevitable newness, a "so long" and a "hello" at the same time.

The first summer post diagnosis I found myself dissociating from how seriously I needed to take my exposure to the sun. I wore a moderate SPF level of sunscreen but continued to wear bikinis and "forgot" to wear a hat. I was overwhelmed by the thought that I would lose pieces of my identity, and I could not acknowledge the reality of how the sun could be a danger to me. I was terrified. All I could see was the loss without being able to see any of the other possibilities, so I checked out. Unfortunately, I had to learn the hard way that not only was I not going to lose my identity, but I was also not going to be able to will or to dissociate the reality away. Not surprisingly, I broke out in red itchy blotches all over my body, which were unbearable, I was exhausted all of the time, my hair was falling out, and my joints were in great pain. I needed to take a round of steroids to get my immune system back under control.

It took my body speaking loudly and clearly to bring into my awareness that which I had been dissociated from. I do not think anything else would have done it. After that summer I had to confront what I needed to do to protect myself. I didn't like it, but I knew that I needed to do it. It took about five years, and a lot of therapy, before I felt comfortable in my new beach wardrobe. Before that, I was embarrassed when going to the beach and I felt really angry that I had to do all these extra things to protect myself. That is no longer the case. At some point I stopped being preoccupied with what other people would think because I was more concerned with how I would physically feel. I also realize retrospectively that eventually I had integrated into my identity the experience of the "protective routine" as a new part of me. Even more comforting, I now also recognize that even though I lost the carefreeness that I had while on the beach, I never really lost the beach-carefree part of myself.

> "Health is the ability to stand in the spaces between realities without losing any of them. This is what I believe self-acceptance means and what creativity is really all about—the capacity to feel like one self while being many."
> —P.M. BROMBERG (1993)

IDENTITY AND SELF-STATES

Many people who live with an **autoimmune disease**, like me, struggle with fears of losing their identity post diagnosis. As discussed in Chapter 3, people living with these diseases experience a range of losses, therefore it is not surprising that they would anticipate another loss. Identity is tied to many aspects of daily life that may be disrupted by the disease. For example, a person's identity may be deeply tied to their profession or to their athletic abilities. Someone may feel that if they need to step away from their job or from their sport, their identity will be lost, much like the way that I felt when I could no longer bask in the joys of the beach in the way that I used to.

Bromberg (1993) points out that most people take for granted that their identity or self-representation is a single and unified thing, but that in fact this is an illusion. Bromberg describes how people have a number of discrete, typically overlapping schemata of who they are, which are made up of self-other configurations called self-states. Our experience of ourselves consists of relatively separate self-states which are each coherent in their own right; however, we also have an experience of being a unitary self. My understanding and use of Bromberg's term "unitary self" is to describe what is meant when discussing the experience of "identity." According to Bromberg, when the illusion of unity is traumatically threatened, a person may feel overwhelmed and may be unable to process the experience, oftentimes dissociating from the experience all together.

This is what happened to me when I dissociated from the reality that I could no longer be at the beach in the way that I used to. I thought that part of me, that self-state which encapsulated all of the relationships with people, the sea and sea life, and the beach itself would be gone. I was terrified that I would no longer be the same person that I always saw myself as. Bromberg (1993) believes that every psychotherapy patient starts out with the same illogical wish to stay the same while at the same time changing. He asserts that it is the clinician's job to contribute to preserving the illusion—meaning the illusion of one unitary self. This is our task as mental health professionals who work with patients living with **autoimmune diseases**. It is our job to help our patients adapt to the inevitable changes, including concrete ones but also changes to our various self-other configurations, while still maintaining a sense of a unitary self. So how do we do that?

When a person with an **autoimmune disease** is frightened about losing their identity, what they may not realize is that it doesn't have to mean that the particular part of their self that is associated with a functional loss disappears. If we think about our unitary self or our identity as a shifting configuration of multiple self-states, which are always present but sometimes in the foreground and other times in the background, we can understand that we never really lose those parts of ourselves. The carefree, beach-loving part of me is a self-state that was at the foreground when I was on the beach but was (and is) still always there with me and is a part of me even when I am not at the beach. It is just not in the foreground. That part of the self and the self-other configurations that it consists of will still exist as a self-state, but it will be experienced in a different way. It may be a part of the self that will present in the foreground less frequently or it may find expression through new platforms.

For example, that carefree part of me, my beach self-state, is very present when I sing. Although I am not at the beach, that feeling of carefreeness and the relationships that I internalized while on the beach as a younger person, is very much in the foreground when I am singing. The expression and platform of that carefreeness has changed, meaning the beach is no longer the medium for it, but that part of myself is still very much there. It took work for me to truly believe this, but again that is the task—to accept the contradiction of staying the same while changing.

WORD TO THE WISE

Here is the bottom line. Our patients' sense of a unitary self may feel threatened as functional losses begin to come with their illnesses (e.g. loss of profession, movement, energy). It is important for us mental health professionals to remember that if we think of identity in terms of multiplicity or multiple self-states, then this idea of an identity with a capital I is an illusion anyway. Our job is to help our patients maintain this illusion of a unitary self while also helping them to become aware of and get to know their multiple self-states intimately. Then our patients will be able to see that the beach self-state, for example, was more than just about the beach, but rather is a matrix of relationships that now live independently and is associated with an affective experience of carefreeness. If we can help our patients identify their own self-states, understand the self-other configurations that make them up, and describe the affective experiences that are associated with them, then we can help our patients to see that these parts of them can still exist in some form even though their lives have functionally changed.

For example, I may have lost the feeling of carefreeness at the beach, but the associations I have to my friends, to the feeling of carefreeness, and to the sensory experiences of the beach still exist and are in the foreground when I sing, especially when I sing in Greek. We can work with our patients to help them reconnect to the parts of themselves that they feared that they had lost. Additionally, we help them to recognize and come to know the new self-states that have emerged in relation to their illness. This is "standing in the spaces between realities without losing any of them" (Bromberg, 1993, p. 166). This is the irony of how we maintain the illusion of a unified identity by recognizing and acknowledging the multiple old and new parts of our selves that are born from the matrix of our relationships and experiences as living beings. Helping patients to "stand in the spaces" requires that we address patients' dissociation delicately but directly. As clinicians, we may or may not always know what is being unacknowledged by the patient—what is being dissociated. For example, I talked about what my doctor told me about how sun exposure is dangerous for me; however, I could have unconsciously omitted that information when talking to my therapist or anyone for that matter, and that would have been me dissociating.

Therefore, step one is figuring out what is being dissociated. The "what" can take the form of dissociated content, like "forgetting to wear a hat," or it could take the form of dissociated affect, like saying, acting, and convincing yourself that you are "fine" covering up at the beach when you are really sad about it.

After dissociation is acknowledged, then we can start to slowly, but intimately, get to know the parts of the client that they fear are being lost due to the change that they are struggling with, and the parts of the client that are newly being formed. We can start by asking questions and strive to develop the client's curiosity about that which has been dissociated, while being very attuned to shifts in the client's affect and feeling of safety. Simple questions such as, "Would you say that (insert activity or experience) was a very big part of your life? What kind of feelings did you experience when you did that activity? Do you ever feel those feelings when you are not doing that activity? and who would you do that activity with?" can go a long way in helping a clinician get to know the parts of the client that the client may fear they are losing.

A very big part of this process also includes acknowledging the very real losses that come with living with an **autoimmune disease** and helping the patient to mourn them. We must be very careful not to minimize the losses while exploring self-states after a patient has had a particular functional or concrete loss. It is important to strive for a "both and" approach where we help the patient acknowledge and mourn the functional or concrete loss but also work to help the patient find the self-other configurations and affective experiences associated with that self-state in their present life.

THAT'S NEW!

Living with an **autoimmune disease** creates various affective experiences in relation to both self and other, which can contribute to the development of new parts of the self. Some of these new self-states will be unique to the individual person but there are also some states that are frequently experienced by people who live with **autoimmune diseases**. Some examples of states frequently experienced by those living with **autoimmune diseases**, which will be discussed are, the "anticipatory self-state," the "fearful self-state," the "spark of hope," the "relieved," the "transcendent self-state," the "defeated," the "cared for," and the "abandoned self-state." As will be described, these self-states are more than just moments of a specific feeling. They are moments of experience, infused with affect and associated with particular self-other configurations. For example, the "relieved self-state" is not just a feeling of relief, it comes with so much more. Let's explore these self-states.

The "anticipatory self-state" is associated with the fear of "what may come." It includes a feeling of looming anxiety about something that may or may not occur and involves a dynamic where another person holds an enormous amount of power. When a person living with **autoimmune disease** is in this state, they will likely be distracted, ruminating on the thing that may or may not come, and may ask repeated questions of another person who they perceive to have some knowledge that they themselves do not have. It is very difficult to be attuned to others' experiences while in the "anticipatory self-state" as the patient is likely preoccupied with their own situation. This self-state will most likely appear when waiting for the results of a test. In this scenario, the doctor is the one who holds the power of knowing the test result before the patient does. The patient may be struggling to think about anything other than what the test result will be, as well as the various implications of a particular result, and may also repeatedly check their online portal or call the doctor's office. This state may also present itself when a patient hears news about a change in another patient's health. It may also emerge in anticipation of a medical appointment.

Unlike the "anticipatory self-state," the "fearful self-state" involves a feeling of fear about something that is happening in the present moment as opposed to anticipating something that may or may not happen in the future. The "fearful self-state" is associated with an intense feeling of terror, may include crying or panic attacks, and may involve dissociation from the prospect of hope. While in this self-state, people may find themselves experiencing a great dependence on others for comfort, while also fearing that nobody else can help them. The "fearful self-state" may be in the foreground when a patient receives their diagnosis. For example, they may hear the words, "You have an **autoimmune disease**," and may immediately feel terror and a disconnect from anything else that their doctor is telling them. In this moment, the person may want to have a loved one with them but will likely not feel relieved by their loved one's gestures or words until this state is no longer in the foreground. This state may also present during severe flares, during hospitalization, or when receiving unwanted outcomes of test results.

The "spark of hope" state does not usually last very long but emerges from time to time when a patient receives good news. Mariah went for her regular check-in appointment with her rheumatologist following her routine labs. Her doctor told her that they had reviewed the results of her labs, and they were very much improved from the previous labs. Hearing this, Mariah felt hopeful, she couldn't stop smiling all day, she felt very thankful toward her doctor, and was full of energy the rest of the day. She wanted to tell her partner and was eager to be social that evening. The "spark of hope" state is associated with an experience of hopefulness that one's health will improve, feelings of elation and joy, gratitude, and a desire to connect with others, as others are perceived as helpful. Although this state usually presents when receiving positive news, it can also enter the foreground at times when another is experienced as being helpful. The "spark of hope" is different from being a generally optimistic person.

It is a state that can present itself in all people regardless of their general attribution style, and it is brought into the foreground by a particular experience that involves another person providing help or perceived help.

The phrase "a breath of fresh air" comes to mind when I think of the self-state of "the relieved." It is that moment of finding a breath after having held it for so long, that includes an experience of muscle relaxation, calm, and a sense of safety. As mentioned earlier, however, this state is not just a feeling of relief but an experience of self-other configurations, associations, and affect. In this state, one's relationship with others is one of connection, as the patient has the mental space to attend to others. There is often an excitement to share what one is relieved about, and feelings of joy. Usually, people will experience a shift from the "anticipatory self-state" to "the relieved" state, as "the relieved" state typically emerges when procedures, surgeries, stronger medications, or negative test results are avoided following a period where the patient is waiting to learn what their next steps will be.

After living with an **autoimmune disease** for some time, many people begin to accept and make meaning of their condition and sometimes even feel gratitude for some of the experiences that come with living with the illness. This is what I call the "transcendent self-state."

Ariadne, a young woman in her late twenties diagnosed with lupus, said to me, "Lupus has given me a gift. I don't wish to have an illness but living with lupus has given me wisdom that most people my age do not have. I really value my life and see how precious it is. I think this is something only old people usually have." As a result of living with her illness, Ariadne is aware of a new state when she feels aware of what is valuable in life and what is worth worrying about, and she feels a tremendous appreciation for life. Some people who live with **autoimmune disease** never develop this state, and as will be explored in Chapter 7, it is our job as mental health professionals to help our clients connect to moments where this state may be experienced. The "transcendent state" is associated with a feeling of acceptance, dignity, empowerment, and agency. When this state is in the foreground, relationships with others are experienced as precious and there is an honesty and directness in how the person living with the illness communicates with others about their needs.

The antithesis of the "transcendent state" is the "defeated state." People who live with **autoimmune disease** tend to shift into this state during prolonged periods of flaring. This state is associated with having tried multiple prescription medications, sometimes holistic treatments, vitamins, supplements, various physical therapies and bodywork treatments, and lots of rest, without successful relief of the flare up. Feelings that are present during this state are often despair, hopelessness, and detachment from others. People may understand their experience as one that cannot be understood by anyone else, even perhaps by other people who are also living with an **autoimmune disease**.

Jana is on a special diet because of her Hashimoto's disease. She doesn't eat dairy or gluten. Jana is used to having to inspect restaurant menus before venturing out or making sure to eat at home before visiting another's home. She doesn't take for granted that there will be something that she can eat if she is eating outside her home. Jana felt very cared for when prior to her friend's birthday party, her friend contacted her and informed her of the birthday dinner menu and asked her if this would be something Jana could eat. The "cared for" state is so much more than the feeling of being cared for. It is associated with an experience of being able to relax and trust that one's needs will be attended to or that requests will not be ignored. Relationships with others are experienced as safe and caring. The person living with the illness does not experience themselves as a burden on others and relationships feel secure.

The "abandoned" self-state is the antithesis of the "cared for" self-state. This state usually emerges after a person living with **autoimmune disease** has an experience where their needs that come with living with the illness are neglected or ignored. For example, if Jana's friend did not call to see if Jana could eat anything on her birthday menu, and if she did not serve any gluten and dairy free options, Jana may have shifted into the "abandoned" state. When this self-state is in the foreground, the person living with the illness may feel like they are on their own, and may experience thoughts such as, "I can't expect other people to remember my needs." Relationships with others may be thought of as limited in terms of providing empathy because of the belief that others will not be able to hold in mind the needs of the person living with the illness. Feelings associated with this state are anger, frustration, disappointment, and apathy.

The aforementioned self-states, just like any other self-state, will fluctuate from being in the foreground to being in the background of a person's experience. Not all of these self-states will be a significant part of every person who lives with **autoimmune disease**, and people may also have new self-states as part of their journey of living with an **autoimmune disease** that have not been discussed in this chapter. Some feelings that are part of these self-states that emerge when living with an **autoimmune disease** were likely part of a person's experience prior to being diagnosed with their disease. However, what makes these states different from experiences the person had before being diagnosed is the self-other configurations and associations that come along with the feelings that emerge in each state. These associations and self-other configurations are now a new part of the person's life and will always be, whether in the background or in the foreground of the person's experience.

ON SHAKY GROUND

"Why would they stay in a relationship with me?" "How can I commit to plans if I don't know how I am going to feel that day?" "I might as well avoid socializing." "Damn it, why won't you help me?" "I need you." "Leave me alone." "I don't need your help." These are some common questions and statements that people who live with **autoimmune diseases** often make. As discussed earlier in the chapter on interpersonal relationships, people living with **autoimmune disease** often worry about how the people in their lives will react to the needs that come from living with their illness. It is understandable that there could be a tremendous amount of anxiety about the security of relationships when living with an **autoimmune disease**. A consequence of this is that a person's feelings and behaviors may resemble that which is consistent with an insecure attachment style (anxious and ambivalent specifically), which may manifest as anxiety about losing or being rejected by loved ones, ambivalence about intimacy in relationships, suppressing emotions, and ambivalence about dependency on others.

One may ask, understandably, "What do you mean by 'these feelings and behaviors may resemble' an insecure attachment style? Maybe the person actually *has* an insecure attachment style." Some of these patients may indeed have an insecure attachment style and this is something that as clinicians we are able to assess as we learn about the patient's history and early relationships with their caregivers. However, what is of importance when working with patients who live with **autoimmune disease** is that even patients who have secure attachments throughout their lives may suddenly appear to have insecure attachments. Patients themselves are often aware of their own behaviors and feelings that seem new and unfamiliar to them and frequently do not like having these behaviors and feelings but may also believe that they are necessary. Let's explore an example of what this may look like.

Cara had grown up in a stable and loving family. She was very close to both her parents and grandparents, who played a large role in her upbringing. She had a long term high school boyfriend and a number of close friends, and overall felt a sense of security in her relationships.

Although very independent, Cara was always able to ask directly for what she needed from the people in her life and would often get frustrated when people were indirect about their needs. She felt confident in her relationships and never saw herself as someone overly preoccupied with potential rejection from others.

Things changed for Cara when she was diagnosed with a very severe case of systemic lupus while she was on a temporary work assignment, far away from her hometown, her friends, and her family. This illness dramatically changed her life in that she felt chronically exhausted, experienced debilitating pain, and at times found herself struggling to stand or walk. The illness also altered the way she viewed and felt about relationships and subsequently changed her behavior in respect to how she engaged relationally with others. She worried a lot about being "too needy" and being a burden on others, she became reluctant to directly ask for what she needed, and she anticipated that any man she dated would reject her once they learned about her medical needs.

Many painful experiences contributed to changes in Cara's feelings and behaviors, beginning with the drastic physical limitations that came with her illness and continuing with hurtful and disappointing encounters with others. The series of experiences that Cara understands as having created her new insecurities involved multiple interactions with the boyfriend she was dating when she was diagnosed. Cara described how he didn't seem to grasp the gravity of her diagnosis and would make comments that made Cara feel badly for not being able to participate in social activities and at times not able to engage in sex. Rather than making an effort to figure out how to include Cara in social plans or find a way to adapt so that both their needs were met, her boyfriend stopped inviting her to social events and told her that she was "too fragile" to be around his friends. For many months, Cara blamed herself for the conflict in their relationship and was worried about his disapproval until he ended the relationship with her.

Following this relationship, Cara was extremely anxious about dating and believed that there wouldn't be a man that could handle her diagnosis. Her experience with her previous boyfriend also created insecurities in her relationships where there weren't any before, and Cara was frequently anxious about whether she had offended others, despite there not being a reason for another to be offended.

WORD TO THE WISE

Cara is someone who had a secure attachment style and yet her experiences living with systemic lupus impacted her so tremendously that for almost a decade post diagnosis she presented as someone with an anxious attachment style. If someone with a solidly secure attachment style can be shaken this much, imagine patients who are starting from a baseline of insecure attachment.

You may find a prospective patient in a dysregulated state, having mood swings (which also may be worsened by certain medications like steroids), and at times presenting with behaviors and thoughts that resemble a personality disorder. Some patients may indeed have a comorbid personality disorder; however, as discussed in earlier chapters many patients will have clinical depression and anxiety, but most patients will not have a personality disorder, even if at first it may appear to you that they do. After a period of time working with patients who have **autoimmune diseases** (who do not also have a personality disorder), a clinician will be able to recognize that the patients' behaviors, affect, relational dynamics, and thoughts that may signal personality disorder, are manifestations of an already insecure attachment baseline that has been extremely rattled by the trauma, multiple hurts, losses, and relational pain that can come with being diagnosed with such a disease.

Georgia is a middle-aged professional woman who worked many hours and prided herself on her career identity. After her third pregnancy, she developed symptoms of **autoimmune disease** and after several years of medical appointments was subsequently diagnosed with multiple sclerosis. My first encounter with Georgia was jarring. Georgia had called me up in a frantic state, wanting to know how soon I could see her. She spoke very rapidly and loudly as she asked if she should come in for individual therapy or if she should be seen with her husband who she was in high conflict with during that time. She told me how angry she felt with her husband for suggesting that she temporarily take a step back from work to focus on her health. She said that she stopped telling him anything about her health because she "didn't want to hear it from him and that she generally wasn't talking to him right now."

After she shared this information, she demanded to know why I couldn't see her sooner than her present appointment. I let her know that, unfortunately, the time I had offered her was the earliest available time I had. Georgia became quiet and coldly said that she would come in at that time.

When I hung up the phone, I felt myself becoming overwhelmed. I wondered about who Georgia was and how she would act during our sessions. I wondered if she would be emotionally and behaviorally volatile. In what ways would I be the target of her anger? Would she push me away like she did with her husband if I said something she didn't agree with? What I learned as I got to know Georgia is that she has an avoidant attachment style. From a very young age, Georgia had to rely on herself to get her needs met. She had become extremely skilled at getting physical and material needs met but her emotional needs remained unmet well into her adulthood. Georgia has struggled to allow herself to be vulnerable with others and with herself as well. She doesn't trust caring actions, feels like she shouldn't be dependent on others, and can quickly shut down emotionally when hurt.

When Georgia received her diagnosis, it terrified her, forced her into a place of vulnerability, and created a situation in which she would have to depend on others for certain things, like medical care and physical help. Her default style in a situation like this would be to shut down and try to figure things out on her own but again she couldn't do that in this situation, so instead she doubled down on her avoidant behaviors and yelled at her husband, stopped talking to him, stopped talking to me for a few moments when I said I couldn't see her sooner, and refused to reflect on the possibility that she may need to temporarily slow her career down until she was in a better place with her health. Receiving her diagnosis intensified her existing avoidant behaviors and she appeared emotionally labile and very dysregulated, but this was not Georgia's baseline. After spending several weeks with Georgia and exploring her difficulties with being vulnerable and needing help from others, Georgia was a lot calmer. Although still resistant to and frustrated with the need to rely on others, Georgia recognized that this was something that she was going to have to work on.

WORD TO THE WISE

As discussed, being diagnosed and living with an **autoimmune disease** can create massive shifts in how a person perceives themselves and how they feel and behave in relation to others. It is critical that clinicians recognize and retain awareness of all the different ways that a patient's identity has not only seemingly shifted but also how it remains the same, in order to help a patient maintain a sense of a unitary identity. It is similarly important, as in most cases, to avoid jumping to conclusions about patients' attachment styles based on only brief and limited interactions with them. This may seem like an obvious statement, but it is always worth the reminder.

7

TRANSCENDENCE: BEYOND THE ILL

I REMEMBER FEELING ANGRY with my body when I was first diagnosed with lupus because my body no longer felt like my own. My body felt like an agent of this enemy "other"—this illness that was not a part of me, it was unwanted, and it had co-opted my body, wreaking havoc on my life. When you're living with an **autoimmune disease**, it is hard to imagine anything positive or meaningful about it. In fact, even the suggestion of that as a possibility may not even be something that can be entertained. This *can* change! This is a part of what I call "transcendence."

According to the Oxford Dictionary (2024), the definition of transcendence is "the ability to go beyond the usual limits, existence, or experience beyond the normal or physical level." When thinking about **autoimmune disease**, transcendence means going beyond the cognitions, feelings, and behaviors that keep a person stuck in the experience of illness as "other" that only breeds helplessness, and which feels completely uncontrollable. This is not to say that a person who has experienced a state of transcendence actually wants to live with an **autoimmune disease** or that achieving a state of transcendence will eliminate the negatives that come with living with illness.

What this does mean is that a person can push beyond their cognitions, behaviors, and feelings about the illness that have felt fixed, and they can start to connect with an experience of agency, empowerment, and dignity, as well as positives that have come into their life only because of their experience with **autoimmune disease**. They can begin to make meaning of the illness, and the illness becomes incorporated into being a part of the person rather than a controlling "other" that is separate from one's self.

The phrase "it doesn't define you" is something that a person who is living with an **autoimmune disease** may hear often, but the truth is that having an **autoimmune disease** does define a part of a person who is living with it. The good news is that in some ways, a person gets to determine how it defines them. Similar to what was discussed in Chapter 6, new parts or states of a person emerge through the experience of living with illness, and transcendence can be one of these states. Transcendence is the state of learning to live your best life with **autoimmune disease** as part of it.

We know that living with an **autoimmune disease** is an unnatural occurrence. However, this is not to say that there is something wrong with a person who may have such a disease. What it does mean is that it is something that the body does that it is not meant to do. Most people are not in their elderly years when they begin to exhibit symptoms of an **autoimmune disease** or when they are diagnosed. They are not at an age where people are typically aware of how fragile and how short life is, and yet they are forced, by the experience of having an **autoimmune disease**, to confront this reality—again, it is unnatural. This presents an opportunity to transform this experience into wisdom, into meaning, into empowerment, into dignity, and into advocacy. With time and with the help of informed psychotherapy, people who live with **autoimmune diseases** can experience their illness as a part of their self, a part that they can also feel positive about. This is transcendence! Let's now explore some of the constituents that comprise the state of transcendence.

MAKING MEANING

I was diagnosed with lupus when I had just turned 30. I had just come out of my twenties feeling invincible. I was extremely athletic and physically strong, and I believed that I had an entire lifetime to live in a manner not so different from how I was living. It was a rude awakening after my symptoms began to progress and there were days when it was difficult to move myself out of bed or when there were moments that it took effort to walk. These experiences forced me to come face to face with the body's (including my body's) fragility. Even more frightening, when I learned about how lupus can involve organ damage, I had to confront the reality that mortality was not something that only the elderly had to contend with. It is one thing to know this cognitively as a concept. We all know that young people also die or that young people can have fragile bodies. However, it is a completely different experience to live it and to know it from the inside out as a reality beyond the conceptual. This is not something that can be taught but only felt.

Throughout this book, I have discussed the multiple feelings that can accompany living with an **autoimmune disease**, like fear, trauma, depression, shame, and anxiety for example. How can a person living with an autoimmune illness take these feelings and transform them into something that feels positive and meaningful? I remember in the first one or two years after being diagnosed with lupus I was terrified of having organ damage. I remember learning about a young woman in her twenties who ended up in the hospital with kidney failure due to lupus. I thought about how if this could happen to her, it could happen to me. I felt paralyzed by this fear, but I found comfort in writing about it. I found myself writing and writing, and I realized that perhaps other people may have similar feelings or experiences.

I decided to start posting my writing as a blog on the, at the time, popular blogspot.com. There was something meaningful to me about sharing my writing with the world, not only because it felt like I could put my feelings into action, but also because it created a community for me. I received emails from people all over the world commenting on my writing. Some people wrote to tell me how much they related to what I was writing about. Others encouraged me to keep writing because they looked forward to reading what I had to say, and some people just wanted to say hi and connect. This experience was extremely meaningful to me because it was the beginning of the writer part of me that I had not experienced before.

Since then, I have found so much solace in writing and I have discovered that not only do I enjoy writing about various topics, but that writing is also an exercise that is healing to me. It allows me to feel agentic and empowered. I don't know if I would've discovered this part of myself had I not been compelled by the intense feelings of fear that came with my **autoimmune disease**. I did not know what else to do with these feelings, so I wrote.

WORD TO THE WISE

My experience with writing is an example of generativity and creativity that allowed me to make meaning of a very painful and frightening situation. When working with your clients, it may be helpful to brainstorm with them to find a creative activity that they have always wanted to engage in or that they used to engage with in the past. Is there something they might want to create that they could feel a connection to or perhaps even feel proud of? Work with your client to think outside of the box—be creative with them.

This is not exclusive to artistic expressions. It can indeed be things like visual arts or musicality, but creativity can also be any act of generativity that is experienced as new to the person themselves. Perhaps a business idea emerges or a new idea about how to make it possible to travel more frequently despite physical limitations. Generativity and creativity can take infinite forms. However, what creates meaning is that these acts of generativity and creativity are experienced by the client as directly related to living with the **autoimmune disease**. As clinicians, we can work with our clients to identify and engage with these specific acts that provide this meaning. Engagement in these acts can create a feeling of agency and empowerment for the person living with the illness.

REDUCTION OF SHAME

"What do I do if I go to the party, and I don't feel well and have to leave? I am so embarrassed that I need to wear all these clothes that cover me up at the beach. I am so ashamed that my hair has fallen out. It is so embarrassing that my muscles tense up and I start to shake. Why can my colleagues work so many more hours without feeling as tired as me? I am sorry that I have to ask the server so many questions about the ingredients in the food." These are just a few of the expressions of shame that people who live with **autoimmune disease** often share. There are many more situations that accompany feelings of shame for people who live with these illnesses. As discussed earlier in this book, shame is a feeling to contend with when living with **autoimmune disease**. It is a difficult feeling to challenge but part of transcendence is finding a way to communicate with the shameful feelings so that they do not persistently interfere with a person's wellbeing.

Annabella is in her mid-twenties and has been living with type I diabetes for a few years now. Although she often felt lonely, she struggled to engage in social events because of feelings of shame about her illness. She worried about her peers noticing her blood glucose monitor and she didn't want attention drawn to her if she felt faint, needed to consume some food or lay down. Annabella had an incident at a party where her blood sugar dropped quickly, and she fainted. Although her friends were very supportive and kind, she felt a lot of shame about her illness and about her body for what she perceived as her body having "failed her." After this incident at the party, Annabella carried a feeling of shame with her every time she was in a social setting, regardless of how she was feeling physically. She experienced having an **autoimmune disease** as something shameful because it could draw unwanted attention to her and cause an unwelcome scene, so she began to isolate herself.

Annabella no longer avoids social situations and no longer associates her illness with shame! This did not happen overnight, but Annabella did embark on a process of slowly reducing feelings of shame around her illness. How did this process begin? A big part of this change occurred when Annabella joined a support group for young people with chronic illnesses. She met people who also live with type I diabetes, as well as others with all sorts of chronic conditions, and she was impressed with how confident some of these folks were. In conversation with some of her peers from the group, Annabella learned that living with an illness or being differently abled is a demographic identity just like any other, like ethnicity, gender, or race. She was able to witness that like other identities, this can also be an identity to be proud of because it is a part of who she is.

Again, this did not happen overnight, but with time Annabella became more comfortable with her illness and what came along with it. Currently when she attends social gatherings, she openly checks her monitor and takes care of her medical needs.

WORD TO THE WISE

Encourage your clients to be as social as possible! Provided they feel safe in a given setting, encourage your clients to be as open about their illness in social settings as they feel that they can. For example, if a client needs to follow a specific diet, recommend that they try to verbalize that out loud in front of others or in restaurants. Suggest to your client that they could benefit from finding peers who struggle with the same or another **autoimmune diseases**. All these actions empower and help a person living with an **autoimmune disease** to feel less alone, less "different" or "other," and can reduce feelings of shame associated with their illness. When a person engages in these actions, they are inevitably in an active dialogue with their shame, acknowledging that it is there but also letting the shame know that it isn't as powerful anymore.

The message mental health practitioners want to communicate to their clients is that to engage in these actions is not shameful but dignified. You want your clients to feel like they have just as much a right to exist in the way that they/their bodies exist as anyone else.

Part of transcendence may also include reduction of shame, specifically around bodily functions, appearance, and physical abilities. As explored earlier in this book, many people who live with **autoimmune diseases** feel shame around what their body cannot do, what it does outside of their control, and/or changes in their appearance due to the illness. Franky, a woman in her mid-twenties, has plaque psoriasis which presents with scaly raised red patches on her elbows extending up her arms and in the back of her head down to the back of her neck. Franky was diagnosed in her early twenties and was very anxious about how this diagnosis would impact her appearance. She was concerned about dating and worried that potential partners would be disgusted by her body. During the first two years post diagnosis, Franky spread a lot of liquid makeup on her psoriasis hoping it would hide the patches of red, raised skin.

As you can imagine, this action did not leave Franky feeling very good about herself, and it reinforced the false narrative that she had something to be ashamed of. After some time and some hard work, Franky's experience of her body shifted, and she no longer carries the same burden of shame around her psoriasis. She has come to confront the myths around what beauty is that cause so many people to suffer, and she recognizes her shame as something fueled by those myths. Franky actively chooses to confront her shame, letting her skin breathe, free from makeup, and she feels empowered as she does so.

WORD TO THE WISE

It is important to work with your clients to identify the ways in which shame about their bodies manifests and impacts their lives. They may not always be so obvious, as in Franky's case. For example, it could be that a person's posture has changed, not because of any anatomical change but because the feeling of shame has made a person recoil into themselves, without the person even realizing it. Perhaps a person speaks less spontaneously in groups than they used to without noticing but upon reflection they realize that they were avoiding drawing attention to themselves.

Help your client to think deeply about any changes in their behavior or interactions and to reflect on the possibility of these changes being related to feelings of shame around their body. Once the impact of body shame has been identified, it can be challenged. By confronting their shame, a client can experience empowerment and dignity. Prior to encouraging a client to confront their shame, it is crucial that the clinician make space for their client to mourn the losses that have come from living with their disease, lest the client feel invalidated.

Techniques that mental health professionals will use to help their clients feel less shame around their bodies will vary depending on the particular circumstances of the client's illness and history. The idea behind the techniques, however, will be similar, with the intention being the fostering of empowerment and dignity. Shame makes a person feel small, want to hide, and powerless compared to others. A person with an **autoimmune disease** may feel incapable, unattractive, and hidden.

Clinicians can encourage their clients to push back against body shame by striving to hide less. We could liken this to an exposure technique except rather than extinguishing anxiety, the goal is to tolerate and ultimately reduce shame. Encourage your client to look in the mirror at the parts of their body that they feel ashamed of. Identify the negative thoughts that the client associates with their body and work with the client to replace them with positive thoughts if possible or neutral thoughts. Suggest your client be mindful of their posture if it is in their control and ask them to try to intentionally change it. Recommend to your client that they attend a situation that they would have typically avoided because of shame related to involuntary movements in their body. Again, these are just some examples and the techniques that you will use with your client may vary. What is most important is to empower your client to challenge shame and the behaviors that accompany it, and to reinforce behaviors that can foster a sense of dignity.

FINDING THE WORDS

So much of the autoimmune experience starts out unsymbolized and without words. People who are newly diagnosed with an **autoimmune disease** may not immediately know what they feel about having a chronic diagnosis. Even if they have a sense of what they may be feeling, it may be difficult to identify their feelings in a particular moment.

Identifying the feelings and finding the words to symbolize them is a process that may take time.

Additionally, as discussed in Chapter 2, much like other forms of trauma, many of the feelings related to receiving this diagnosis may be dissociated and therefore not yet attached to language. Brain fog and difficulties with concentration, both possible symptoms of **autoimmune disease**, can also make it hard for a person living with such disease to identify or describe their experience using words. Not being able to recognize and label what one feels can be experienced as a default state of helplessness or of being "stuck" in a state of confusion. When working with people who have **autoimmune disease** in a psychotherapeutic setting, it is important to remember that people may not initially know how to respond to the question of "what are you feeling?" This may remind you of the relationship between alexithymia and **autoimmune disease** discussed in the research in Chapter 6.

Part of transcendence includes finding the words to name and describe one's experiences and feelings. This allows a person to reflect and think about their experiences and feelings associated with having an **autoimmune disease** in a way that allows for making meaning and for directed action. This component of transcendence is the opposite of helplessness or of a feeling of "stuckness." Finding the words is an active process, something that one engages in that brings clarity and progressively blows away clouds of confusion.

As mental health professionals this is our forte and I do not need to tell you how to go about helping a client to find the words to describe their experiences and feelings. I would however like to share with you a special moment I experienced with a client where dissociation and "stuckness" were opened up and transformed into a feeling of connection and clarity. This is an example of how by simply putting words to what a client may be feeling, an entire experience can be unlocked, and a client may begin to speak more fluidly about something that may previously have felt unnamable.

Sabrina, a woman in her early thirties, has been living with severe lupus since her mid-twenties. She had difficulty expressing her feelings about living with an **autoimmune disease** and often struggled to find the words to describe her experiences. One morning, Sabrina told me that she did not know what to say or how to describe what she was feeling. It was very clear to me that there was something dissociated yet palpably present. She couldn't make eye contact, which was not the norm for her, and she was hunched over her own body. We sat in silence for a good twenty minutes. I wanted to give her space and not rush in too quickly to give her words that may or may not have represented what she was feeling.

As we were sitting in the silence, I began to reflect on my own feelings related to living with **autoimmune disease**. I started to associate with many of the experiences discussed in this book, such as experiences of invisibility, feeling misunderstood by others, worrying about relationships because of the illness, among other concerns. I decided to take the risk of putting some words out there that I thought may resonate with Sabrina. I said, "It can feel really hard to talk about what autoimmune illness feels like when so often you are told that your experience doesn't make sense or is wrong in some way or that it is not real. It's really hard to hold on to words for your experience when over and over what you share doesn't seem to register to others. After a while, maybe the words even start to fade, and I guess it can get really lonely."

Sabrina was making eye contact with me at this point and her eyes were watery. Her body language had changed. She was no longer hunched over. She sat straight up as she started to speak and she said,

"Yes, it is very lonely. I have been feeling so lonely lately because I have been extremely tired and even though Jeremy (Sabrina's husband) and my boss are really nice about it, I don't think they really understand. And my parents think I am not pushing myself enough and that I am making myself more tired. Sometimes I would rather not say anything." Then I said to her, "But it seems like that doesn't feel good either?" Sabrina responded with, "No, it doesn't, but I guess I just feel a little stuck sometimes. It is not really a choice. Sometimes I really don't have the words. I don't even know what is going on sometimes." And now Sabrina was talking, and the moment she put words to her experience, she recognized that she felt a little less lonely.

WORD TO THE WISE

Again, the way in which I approached my interaction with Sabrina is only one of many ways to help a client put words to their experience. Every practitioner will have their unique manner in which they help a client begin to label their feelings. The important thing is that once a client can start naming what they are feeling, they are more present to engage in an action, even if the action is just talking initially, and they can begin to make meaning of their illness. Being able to connect to the words that satisfactorily symbolize one's experience is a big part of transcendence, and psychotherapy can play a very big part in helping a client to do that. Having the words to understand one's experience also allows a client to more easily identify what they need in order to address their feelings. It also clarifies what actions they need to take to go about meeting their needs and it makes it easier for them to more directly communicate these needs to others.

ASSERTIVENESS AND EASE WHEN IT COMES TO NEEDS

A newfound ease with asserting one's needs related to the **autoimmune disease** is also a component of transcendence. This includes communicating and advocating for one's needs to relatives, friends, and colleagues. Oftentimes, as discussed in Chapter 4, people who live with **autoimmune diseases** may feel uncomfortable with requesting accommodations from others, whether it be in a personal or professional capacity. Although at times there are valid reasons for why a person may avoid making certain requests related to their illness, assuming it feels safe to do so, being able to assert one's needs can come with significant benefits. This aspect of transcendence doesn't mean one always receives what they need, but rather it is knowing that their need is valid and that they have the right to ask for it to be met.

This aspect of transcendence is a form of active coping, which is agentic and can contribute to a feeling of empowerment. Similar to how using words to label one's experience can help direct action by allowing for a person to tap into what they are feeling and what they may need, asserting one's needs directs action by taking the steps to acquire those needs. As such, a person is much more likely to have their needs met and to experience an improved quality of life or situation. Unlike with passive forms of coping, asserting one's needs actively challenges feelings of helplessness.

Unfortunately, there are times when a person living with an **autoimmune disease** will assert their needs with respect to their illness and they will receive a hurtful response. Part of transcendence is being able to hold on to the validity and reality of one's needs related to the illness and to continue to advocate for what one needs. Unless the advocacy starts to become more harmful than the lack of accommodation being requested, it is important for a person to believe that they can continue to make the request. For example, many people who live with **autoimmune diseases** feel and perform better at their place of work when they work non-traditional work hours. I have been told by multiple people who live with **autoimmune diseases** that when they initially asked their employer to work alternative hours, they were told that they could not. However, because these people continued to assert this need and to advocate for themselves, they eventually were allowed to work hours that made more sense for them.

WORD TO THE WISE

This aspect of transcendence is a continuation of labeling one's experience with words. As mental health professionals, we listen to the words our clients express once they have connected to them, and we work with our clients to identify what their needs are. We can then role play with them around how they are going to go about asserting these needs. As clinicians, we support our clients in their advocacy by validating the realities of their needs and we encourage them to continue to be active in their coping until they receive what they are looking for. Lastly, we help them to identify when their advocacy is causing them more harm than help. For example, a person may desperately need their partner to help more with domestic chores because they themselves do not have the physical ability to do so. In an effort to feel empowered and a sense of agency, this person continues to advocate for this in their relationship only to be repeatedly disappointed.

In fact, this person's advocacy keeps causing arguments with their partner, leaving them in more distress and with more of a feeling of helplessness than they experienced to begin with. Although initially it would be important for the clinician to validate this person's request and work with them to assert it to their partner, at this point it would be the clinician's responsibility to work with the client to accept that their partner cannot give them what they are asking for. The clinician can then work with the client to find an alternative solution for having this need met, while processing their feelings of hurt and disappointment as well. The clinician can continue to encourage the client to advocate for themselves around other needs and in other situations.

MANAGING DISCRIMINATION

Transcendence includes an ability to manage discrimination around one's illness. This is an incredibly challenging thing to do given that when one is the recipient of discriminatory actions or content, they will likely have an emotional reaction. The person experiencing discrimination may feel unsafe, hurt, shocked, they may dissociate, may become angry, or may feel any other emotion intensely. People may also literally not know how to respond to discriminatory comments. This can result in a feeling of helplessness.

As mental health professionals we can help our clients to process the feelings that emerge following discriminatory encounters, but we can also provide our clients with concrete tips for how to manage these situations. Our most important goal is for our clients to know that if they feel unsafe in any way during such an encounter, they should immediately remove themselves from the situation and find a safe place to go to. In most cases, however, discrimination towards people with **autoimmune diseases** typically comes in the form of microaggressions.

There are certainly people who deliberately intend to exclude those who have **autoimmune diseases** and do not seem concerned about being hurtful. In these cases, the most important thing to do is to avoid these people as much as possible and to report them to the appropriate authority if there is one. If it feels safe, for the sake of feeling agentic and empowered, the person with the **autoimmune disease** may wish to call out the other person's discriminatory behavior but it is important that the person with the **autoimmune disease** does not expect any change to come from this. Clinicians can work with their clients to manage these expectations. If the person living with the **autoimmune disease** chooses to speak out, it should be because it will leave them feeling empowered and not because they are hoping to change the other person's discriminatory perspective.

In most cases of discrimination via microaggressions, the person being discriminatory likely has no idea that they are being hurtful, and in some cases may even believe that they are being kind. For example, a group of employees are planning to go to dinner after a work event and one employee says to another employee who has lupus, "Oh, you don't need to come." The employee who lives with lupus felt hurt and unwanted. However, this was not the intention of the employee who said this. This employee did not realize that they were excluding their colleague. They thought that they were being kind and letting their colleague off the hook because they knew that lupus often makes them feel tired.

In cases like these, where it is not apparent that a person is deliberately trying to discriminate, it could be helpful to acknowledge that the person's intention was not one of harm. In this case for example, the person who has lupus could say, "I know you are trying to be helpful but comments like that actually make me feel excluded" (or whatever it makes the person feel). In other moments, someone may commit a microaggression because they are trying to connect with the person who has an **autoimmune disease**. Using the same example, a person may say to the person who has lupus, "Oh yeah, I really know how it feels because when my kid keeps me up at night, I get tired too." Clearly the fatigue that a person living with lupus experiences is not the same as being tired because of a poor night's sleep.

It is apparent that the intention behind this comment is a positive one, and yet it can still leave the person who has the **autoimmune disease** feeling terrible. In this case the person with lupus can say, "I get that you're trying to relate to my experience but in fact by comparing our experiences it really diminishes the seriousness of my symptoms. I know that wasn't your intention, but it is important for me to explain."

WORD TO THE WISE

Knowing how to manage discriminatory comments and actions is an extension of finding one's words and asserting one's needs. In psychotherapy sessions, we can work with our clients to find the words that they want to assert in these hurtful situations. Sometimes clients will not feel good about how they handled the discriminatory interaction in the moment and will want to explore what they could've said during the interaction that they would've felt better about. If clients are open to this, mental health professionals can encourage their clients to go back and communicate with the person who hurt them. This can give the client another opportunity to communicate in a way that they can then feel good about.

Another component of this aspect of transcendence is advocacy. Many clients may not be interested in advocacy; however, this is an action that not only challenges discrimination against people with **autoimmune diseases** on a large scale, but it is also a powerful form of active coping. Engaging in advocacy is something tangible that a person can do that is within one's control. As discussed throughout this book, people with **autoimmune diseases** are so often confronted with things outside of their control, whether it be physical, emotional, or interpersonal, such as experiencing discrimination from others.

I encourage all practitioners to introduce the idea of advocacy to their clients and to work with their clients to consider whether there is a form of advocacy that would feel helpful to them. The good thing about advocacy is that a person can engage in it as much or as little as they want. No matter how much one participates in advocacy however, it is an opportunity to educate large groups of people about **autoimmune diseases**, including what discriminatory behaviors towards people with **autoimmune diseases** look like. Through advocacy, aspects of what it is like to have an **autoimmune disease** also become a little less invisible.

TRANSCENDENCE

Engaging in advocacy may allow one to make meaning of the struggles related to their illness. This brings us back to the beginning of this chapter in thinking about making meaning. The state of transcendence brings together the making of meaning, the reduction of shame, the finding of words to label one's experiences, the assertion of one's needs, and the management of discrimination. It is easy to see how all these pieces of transcendence interact and build on each other, moving one away from a feeling of helplessness and into a feeling of agency and dignity—making the invisible a bit more visible. Transcendence is empowerment. Transcendence is the way to live one's best life alongside the **autoimmune disease**. Transcendence is finding a way to receive something positive from the **autoimmune disease**, despite the pain and the losses that the illness has brought. Psychotherapy may not be able to cure a person's **autoimmune disease** but through psychotherapy, mental health professionals can play a vital role in helping people find their transcendence.

8

FINAL THOUGHTS

Y OU HAVE NOW made it to the last chapter of *Understanding Auto-immune Disease: A Therapist's Guide to Invisible Illness*. At this point, I imagine that you have noticed that throughout the book the term "**autoimmune disease**" was always fully spelled out and in bold type. This was a very intentional decision. As discussed throughout this book, **autoimmune diseases** have been invisible in so many ways, whether it is the experience of living with an **autoimmune disease**, what these diseases are, funding and research for these diseases, and invisibility within the mental health profession. It felt important to repeatedly and fully name these diseases. The more something is named, the more familiar it becomes, and hopefully the more interested and comfortable people are when talking about them. That was my hope for this entire book. By educating and informing mental health professionals and people in general on the experiences that come with living with **autoimmune disease**, I hope I have contributed to making **autoimmune diseases**, and those who are living with them feel a little less invisible.

Recently, I was having dinner with a colleague who is very well respected in the mental health world. We were talking about this book, and she was surprised to learn how many illnesses are actually **autoimmune diseases**. She also told me that in the last year there had been a noticeable increase of clients coming to her practice who live with **autoimmune disease**. She said that she felt overwhelmed by this because she knows very little about these diseases or how they impact people and their lives. We then discussed the absence of information in the field of mental health on how to work with people who live with **autoimmune diseases**.

Although the information provided in this book is just a beginning, I hope that it can provide a foundational guide for mental health professionals as well as other clinicians who care for those living with **autoimmune diseases**. Chapters 1 through 7 capture what I believe are essential aspects of the **autoimmune disease** experience. It is crucial that mental health professionals who work with clients with these illnesses attend to these components of their clients' experiences. In doing so, clinicians can provide their clients with a space where the clients' experiences may feel visible and even understood.

Being aware of these aforementioned essential aspects allows for understanding and visibility during psychotherapy sessions. Psychotherapy can also provide a space to explore the potential for transcendence—the hope for living one's best life alongside the disease. Keeping in mind the various experiences that comprise the state of transcendence, therapists can work with their clients to create meaning through their illness, reduce shame associated with their illness, find the words to describe their experiences related to their illness, assert their needs, and manage discrimination. The hope is that clinicians will be able to work with their clients to foster feelings of dignity, agency, and empowerment so that they can expand the spaces in their lives in which they feel visible.

Following the release of this book, perhaps additional books, articles, and training will become available. This is my hope. I imagine a day when graduate students learn about **autoimmune diseases** in their academic programs or training sites, or when licensed clinicians can take a continuing education course on this topic. It would be wonderful to have an array of resources to help practitioners work with their clients who live with **autoimmune disease**. This is only the beginning.

Something to look forward to in the near future is a forthcoming companion guide to *Understanding Autoimmune Disease: A Therapist's Guide to Invisible Illness*. This will be a workbook for clients to use either in tandem with their psychotherapeutic treatment or on their own. The workbook chapters will parallel the chapters in *Understanding Autoimmune Disease: A Therapist's Guide to Invisible Illness* and will encourage movement towards transcendence. There will be exercises, reflections, and tips for people who live with **autoimmune disease** that focus on trauma, loss, relationships, identity, coping, among other aspects of the **autoimmune disease** experience. Clinicians can encourage their clients to engage using the activities in the workbook as an adjunct to their psychotherapy sessions. People who live with **autoimmune disease** may also want to share their exercises in the workbook with their caretakers in an effort to increase caretakers' understanding of the **autoimmune disease** experience. It can be a useful tool for working through misunderstandings and strengthening communication.

Caring for a loved one, a patient, or a client who lives with **autoimmune disease** is not something that necessarily comes naturally or is innate. Living with an **autoimmune disease** can at times be extremely difficult, and the same can be said for those who care for people who have these diseases. I have been disheartened by how little information there has been for mental health professionals who work with this population, but I have also been delighted by the desire and hunger of mental health professionals to want to learn more about what it means to live with an **autoimmune disease**. I feel so hopeful and grateful for this increased interest within the mental health field. With this growing curiosity about the experience of living with an **autoimmune disease** comes a growing visibility. Maybe, at least in psychotherapy, the time will come when people who live with these diseases feel no longer invisible.

ACKNOWLEDGMENTS

First, I would like to thank the team at Hatherleigh Press, Andrew Flach, Ryan Tumambing, and Ryan Kennedy, for all of their hard work in making this book a reality and for believing in this project.

I would like to thank my husband John and daughter Athena for all their patience during the process of writing. Their unwavering support was and is invaluable. I could not have done it without them. I love you so much. You are everything.

There are many friends and colleagues whom I would like to acknowledge. A big thank you to Dr. Maria Lechich for her persistent encouragement. I would like to thank Dr. Melanie Suchet and Dr. Karen Starr for helping me believe in myself as a writer. I'd like to acknowledge and thank my esteemed colleagues Dr. Rebeca Scherman, Dr. Natalie Cohen, and Dr. Lisa Orbe'-Austin for their careful reading and feedback on the book, as well as Marisa, whose reaction to the book meant so much to me. Thank you to Dr. Cristina Dorazio for writing such a heartfelt and beautiful preface for this book and for being my dear friend throughout this journey of developing our careers as psychologists.

Thank you Sue Gloor for agreeing to write the foreword for this book and for all the wonderful work you do at the Lupus Foundation of America. Your advocacy for those who feel invisible is an inspiration which I held with me throughout my writing.

Last but not least, I want to acknowledge all of those who have felt unseen and invisible, who have shared their stories with me. This book is for you. I hope it reflects your experience as you'd want it to be known.

**Scan the QR code to visit
author's website.**

ABOUT THE AUTHOR

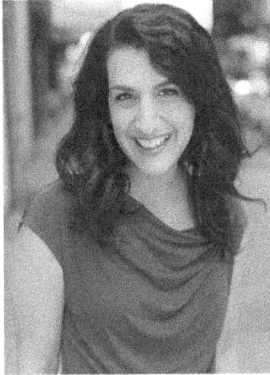

Dr. Nicoletta Skoufalos is a licensed clinical psychologist in private practice in New York City where she works with adults and couples. Dr. Skoufalos received her PhD from Fordham University and trained in multiple New York City hospitals and institutions where she had opportunities to work with patients who had various medical conditions. She currently specializes in working with people who live with chronic medical illnesses, primarily autoimmune diseases and gynecological conditions.

After receiving her license, Dr. Skoufalos began giving talks on the topic of the experience of living with chronic illness and has also had the privilege of participating in speaking engagements, including webinars with the Northeast Division of the Lupus Foundation of America. Dr. Skoufalos has also been interviewed and quoted by various magazines and organizations, such as Women's Health, Health Central, Well Good, Diabetes Forecast, Forbes, the Lupus Foundation of America, Chronic Curve, and others on health and wellness concerns.

Dr. Skoufalos lives with three autoimmune diseases herself and is an active advocate for those living with autoimmune disease. She participates in annual walks to raise money for lupus awareness and for many years has also maintained a blog about the experience of living with chronic illness, available to read on her website GreenTPsychology.com.

REFERENCES

Americans with Disabilities Act (1990). www.ada.gov/law-and-regs/ada/

Autoimmune Association, (2024). Autoimmune.org/resource-center/about-autoimmunity/

Autoimmune Institute (2024). Autoimmuneinstitute.org/resources/autoimmune-disease list/#E

Behkar, A., Garmaroudi, G., Nasimi, M., et al. (2022). Assessing quality of life in patients with autoimmune bullous diseases using the Persian version of Treatment of Autoimmune Bullous Disease Quality of Life Questionnaire finds similar effects in women as men. International Journal of Women's Dermatology, 8 (1).

Bookwalter, D.B., Roenfeldt, K.A., LeardMann, C.A., Kong, S.Y., Riddle, M.S., & Rull, R.P., (2020). Posttraumatic stress disorder and risk of selected autoimmune diseases among U.S. military personnel. BMC Psychiatry, 20: 23.

Booth, S., Price, E., & Walker, E. (2018). Fluctuation, invisibility, fatigue—the barriers to maintaining employment with systemic lupus erythematosus: results of an online survey. Sage Journals, 27 (14).

Bromberg, P. M. (1993). Shadow and substance: A relational perspective on clinical process. Psychoanalytic Psychology, 10 (2), pp. 147-168.

Carruthers, B.M., van de sande, M.I., De Mierleir, K.L., et al., (2011). Myalgic encephalomyelitis : International consensus criteria. Journal of International Medicine, 270 (4), pp. 327-338.

Chang, R., Chen, T., Wang, S-I., et al., (2023). Risk of autoimmune disease in patients with COVID-19: A retrospective cohort study. EClinical Medicine, 56.

Conceicao, C.T.M., Meinao, I.M., Bombana, J.A., & Sato, E.I., (2019). Psychoanalytic 121 psychotherapy improves quality of life, depression, anxiety, and coping in patients with systemic lupus erythematosus: a controlled randomized clinical trial. Advanced Rheumatology, 59 (1), 4.

Freud, S. (1896). The standard edition of the complete psychological works of Sigmund Freud.

Ge, X-L., Li, S-Z., Wang, W., & Zuo, Y-G., (2020). A report of multiple autoimmune syndrome: Pemphigus vulgaris associated with several immune-related diseases after thymectomy. Indian Journal of Dermatology, 65 (4), pp. 320-322.

Greenfield, J., Hudson, M., Vinet, E., et al. (2017). A comparison of health related quality of life across four systemic autoimmune rheumatic diseases. The Public Library of Science, 12 (12).

Gupta, M.A., Vujcic, B., & Gupta, A.K. (2017). Dissociation and conversion symptoms in dermatology. Clinics in Dermatology, 35 (3), pp. 267-272.

Hoffman, D.E. & Tarzian, A.J., (2001). The girl who cried pain: A bias against women in the treatment of pain. The Journal of Law, Medicine, and Ethics, 28 (s4), pp. 13-27.

Johns Hopkins Medicine (2024). www.pathology.jhu.edu/autoimmune/prevalence/

Lee, B., Holt, E.W., Wong, R.J., et al., (2018). Race/ethnicity is an independent risk factor for autoimmune hepatitis among the San Francisco underserved. Autoimmunity, 51 (5), pp. 258-264.

Lumley, M.A, Neely, L.C., & Burger, A.J. (2007). The assessment of alexithymia in medical settings: Implications for understanding and treating health problems. Journal of Personality Assessment, 89 (3), pp. 230-246.

Lupus Foundation of America (2024). Lupus.org/resources/lupus-facts-and-statistics

Lupus Foundation of America (2024). Lupus.org/resources/what-is-lupus

Lupus Research Alliance (2023). Lupus research alliance honors Carola Vinuesa, MD, PhD, for discovering a specific gene variant that causes lupus in some patients. www.LupusResearch.org.

Macarenco, M.M., Opariuc-Dan, C., & Nedelcea, C. (2021). Childhood trauma, dissociation, alexithymia, and anger in people with autoimmune diseases: A mediation model. Child Abuse and Neglect, 122.

Marks, D.F., Murray, M., & Estacio, E.V. (2018). Health psychology: Theory, research, and practice, 5th edition. Sage Publications.

Masson, M.B.. (1984). The Assault on Truth: Freud's Suppression of the Seduction Theory. New York: HarperCollins.

McNamara, L. & Kemper, K. (2011). If you have to wear an ugly dress, learn to accessorize: Guidance, inspiration, and hope for women with lupus, scleroderma, and other autoimmune illnesses. Wheatmark.

Mikulik, M., (2023). Global autoimmune disorders spending from 2011 to 2023. Statista. www.statista.com/statistics.com/statistics/1233691/autoimmune-treatment spend-worldwide/

Miller, F.W. (2023). The increasing prevalence of autoimmunity and autoimmune diseases: an urgent call to action for improved understanding, diagnosis, treatment, and prevention. Current Research in Immunology, 80.

National Institute of Health (2024). National Library of Medicine. www.nlm.nih.gov

Navarette-Navarette, N., Peralta-Ramirez, M.I., Sabio-Sanchez, J.M., Coin, M.A., Robles Ortega, H., Hidalgo-Tenorio, C., Ortego-Centeno, N., Callejas-Rubio, J.L., & Jimenez Alonso, J., (2010). Efficacy of cognitive-behavioral therapy for the treatment of chronic stress in patients with lupus erythematosus: a randomized controlled trial. Psychosomatic Psychotherapy, 79 (2), pp. 107-115.

Nelson. J.L., (2002). Microchimerism and human autoimmune diseases. Sage Journals Rare Disease Collection, 11 (10).

O'Rourke, M.O., (2022). The invisible kingdom: Reimagining chronic illness. Riverhead Books: New York.

Pothemont, K., Quinton, S., Jayoushe, M., et al., (2021). Patient perspectives of medical trauma related to inflammatory bowel disease. Journal of Clinical Psychology in Medical Settings, 29, 596-607.

Ramey, S. (2020), The Lady's Handbook for her Mysterious Illness. Doubleday: New York.

Roberts, M.H. & Erdei, E., (2019). Comparative United States autoimmune disease rates for 2010-2016 by sex, geographic region, and race. Autoimmunity Reviews, 19 (1).

Rose, J.A. (2020). The role of implicit bias and culture in managing and navigating healthcare. Hospital for Special Surgery, www.hss.edu/conditions_role-implicit bias-culture-managing-navigating-healthcare.asp.

Sarno, J. (2006) The divided mind: The epidemic of mindbody disorders. Harper Perennial.

Sharma, C. & Bayry, J., (2023). High risk of autoimmune disease after COVID-19. Nature Reviews Rheumatology, 19, pp. 399-400.

Shigesi, N., Kvaskoff, M., Kirtley, S., et al., (2019). The association between endometriosis and autoimmune diseases: A systematic review and meta-analysis. Human Reproduction Update, 25 (4), pp 486-503.

Shomon, M.J., (2002). Living well with autoimmune disease: What your doctor doesn't tell you…that you need to know. Collins Publishing: New York.

Shrivastava, S., Naik, R., Suryawanshi, H., & Gupta, N. (2019). Microchimerism: A new concept. Journal of Oral Maxillofac Pathology, 23 (2), p. 311.

Sloane, M., Wincup, C., Harwood, R., et. al, (2023). Prevalence and identification of neuropsychiatric symptoms in systemic autoimmune rheumatic diseases: An international mixed methods study. Rheumatology, 63 (5), pp. 1259-1272.

Song, S. & Jason. L.A. (2005). A population-based study of chronic fatigue syndrome (CFS) experienced in differing patient groups: An effort to replicate Vercoulen et al. 's model of CFS. Journal of Mental Health,14:277–289.

Sunnquist, M., (2016). A reexamination of the cognitive-behavioral model of chronic fatigue syndrome: Investigating the cogency of the model's behavioral pathway. College of Science and Heath Theses and Dissertations, Fall 11-22.

Tesch, F., Ehm, F., Vivirito, A., et al., (2023). Incident autoimmune diseases in association with SARS-CoV-2 infection: a matched cohort study. Clinical Rheumatology, 42 (10), 2905-2914.

Thomas Jr., D.E. (2023). The lupus encyclopedia : A comprehensive guide for patients and health care providers, 2nd edition. Johns Hopkins University Press: Baltimore.

United States Census Bureau (2019). www.census.gov/data/ tables/2019/demo/wealth/wealth-asset-ownership.html

United States Department of Health and Human Services (2024). www.Healthcare.gov/health-care-law-protections/grandfathered-plans/

United States Department of Labor (2025). www.dol.gov/agencies/odep/ada/MythsandFacts

Vercoulen JH, Swanink CM, Galama JM, et al., (1998). The persistence of fatigue in chronic fatigue syndrome and multiple sclerosis: Development of a model. Journal of Psychosomatic Research 45: 507–517.

Wessely, S., Butler, S., Chalder, T., & David, A. (1991). The cognitive behavioural management of the post-viral fatigue syndrome. In: Jenkins R, Mowbray J, editors. Post-viral fatigue syndrome. Chichester: John Wiley & Sons;. pp. 305–334.

Wessely S, David A, Butler S, et al., (1989). Management of chronic (post-viral) fatigue syndrome. The Journal of the Royal College of General Practitioners, 39: 26–29.

Wilshire, C., Kindlon, T., Mathees, A., & McGrath, S., (2017). Can patients with chronic fatigue syndrome really recover after graded exercise or cognitive behavioral therapy? A critical commentary and preliminary re-analysis of the PACE trial. Fatigue: Biomedicine, Health, and Behavior, 5 (1), pp. 43-56.

Yildirim, A., Boysan, M., & Cilinger, V. (2020). Associations between sleep quality, severity of dissociation, pathological worry, and functional impairment in multiple sclerosis: A case control study. Düşünen Adam: Journal of Psychiatry and Neurological Sciences, 33(1), 29–39.

Need CE credits? Scan the QR code.

For continuing education credits,
visit Hatherleigh.com.